治癌实录 3

晚期癌症·康复延年纪实

资深中西医结合治癌专家力作
呈现多种不同癌症的真实治疗病案
全面展示中西医结合治癌的实际效果

吴 锦　吴宇光　王 俊◎著

中国科学技术出版社
·北京·

图书在版编目（CIP）数据

治癌实录 . 3, 晚期癌症·康复延年纪实 / 吴锦，吴宇光，王俊著 . — 北京 : 中国科学技术出版社 , 2019.5

ISBN 978-7-5046-7356-5

Ⅰ . ①治… Ⅱ . ①吴… ②吴… ③王… Ⅲ . ①癌—中西医结合—诊疗 Ⅳ . ① R73

中国版本图书馆 CIP 数据核字 (2019) 第 037925 号

策划编辑	焦健姿　王久红	
责任编辑	焦健姿	
装帧设计	长天印艺	
责任校对	龚利霞	
责任印制	李晓霖	

出　　版	中国科学技术出版社
发　　行	中国科学技术出版社发行部
地　　址	北京市海淀区中关村南大街 16 号
邮　　编	100081
发行电话	010-62173865
传　　真	010-62173081
网　　址	http://www.cspbooks.com.cn

开　　本	710mm×1000mm　1/16
字　　数	179 千字
印　　张	16
版　　次	2019 年 5 月第 1 版
印　　次	2019 年 5 月第 1 次印刷
印　　刷	北京威远印刷有限公司
书　　号	ISBN 978-7-5046-7356-5 / R·2371
定　　价	35.00 元

為吳錦教授題詞

中西結合繼往開來

攻癌降魔造福社會

鄭耀宗 教授

中国科学院院士、香港大学前校长　郑耀宗教授题词

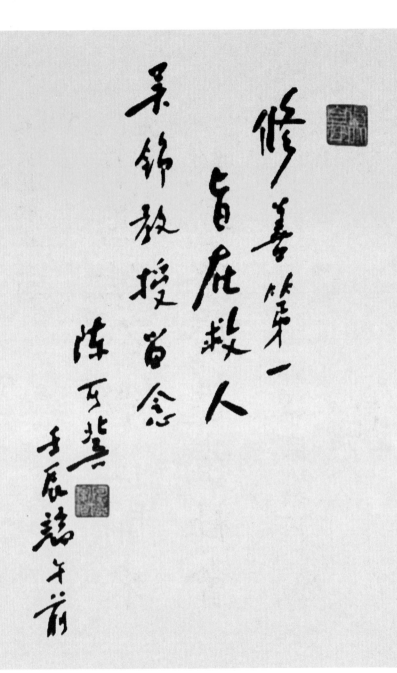

修善第一
旨在救人

采锦教授留念
陈可冀

壬辰端午前

中国科学院院士　陈可冀教授题词

為吳錦教授題詞

中西結合
造福人羣

周肇平 教授

香港中西医结合学会创会会长，香港大学医学院前院长　周肇平教授题词

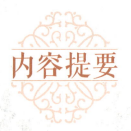

内容提要

　　本书是治癌实录系列的第三部作品，是一部有关晚期癌症治疗的经验集。作者吴锦教授为资深中医药治疗癌症专家，她将自己从事中医药抗癌工作的亲身经历与智慧融会到书中，介绍了她对癌症预防、治疗等方面的看法，以及有关防癌、治癌的基本知识。作者以深入浅出、通俗易懂的写作手法，对生命修复抗癌中医药治疗癌症的原则及方法做了全面论述，并附有大量真实病案。书中病案均保留有原始病历及各种检查报告，同时给出了治疗原则与治疗方案，诊断明确，病例真实，效果确凿，特此公开以鼓励其他患者，特别是晚期癌症患者。希望本书的出版能为更多癌症患者开启抗癌新篇章。

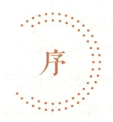

序

　　因为人口老龄化，生活方式（特别是饮食习惯）的变化和环境污染等原因，癌症病发率一直呈上升趋势。现代医学治癌在外科手术、放射治疗和化学治疗等领域都有不少发展。近年，更出现了靶向治疗等新治癌方法。然而，临床效果却不尽如人意。生存质量亦因为放疗、化疗的不良反应大打折扣。因此，许多癌症患者，在经西医确诊以后，会在癌症治疗和康复的各个阶段，自行寻求中医或中西结合治疗，以改善治疗成效和生活质量。

　　我和吴锦教授于多年前就开始在香港中西医结合学会合作，共同促进中西医结合事业在香港的发展。吴教授学问渊博，医术精湛，对促进中西医结合和改善医疗制度充满热忱，对香港中医药发展和中西医结合学会的工作贡献良多。在临床工作方面，吴教授经验丰富，治疗效果显著，特别在癌症的中西医结合治疗方面深受香港广大的癌症患者信任。有感于个人精力有限，无法满足众多患者的需求，吴教授遂将多年的临床经验结合自己在中西医学上的广博知识，以深入浅出的笔触编集成新书，希望能够将一些重要的防癌、治癌和康复、调理的信息广泛传播，让更多的癌症患者受惠。

本书主要系统地介绍了中医治疗癌症的概念和特点，以及中医治疗与西医外科手术、放疗和化疗在癌症不同阶段，在时间上和性质上的不同治法。当中非常清楚地论述了通过中医在"扶正"和"驱邪"两种主要手段上与西医治疗方法的巧妙配合，加强患者和中、西医三方面在治疗的时序和方法方面的默契，从而取得更好的临床效果的过程。此外，吴教授更引用了多种不同晚期癌症的成功治疗案例，让读者可以透过真实病例更好地体会生命修复治癌方法的实际情况和具体成效。

因此，我真诚地向广大癌症患者及其家属、负有临床治癌职务的中西医护人员和对癌症防治有兴趣的朋友推荐吴锦教授的这本新书。

祝大家身体健康！

高永文 GBS, JP
香港防癌会主席
香港中西医结合学会前会长
香港食物及卫生局前局长

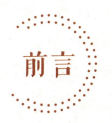

前言

　　癌症是全球最严重的疾病之一，根据世界卫生组织（WHO）2018年最新报道，指出全球癌症发病率和死亡率仍呈迅速上升趋势。世界卫生组织公布的数据表明，全球每年约有880万人死于癌症，占全球每年死亡总人数近六分之一。每年有1400多万新发癌症病例，预计到2030年，这一数字将增加到2100多万。

　　当前主流医学治疗癌症的手段主要是化疗、放疗、手术和靶向抗癌药物等。然而，治疗未必理想和有效，患者往往在经受治疗的痛苦后，仍会发生癌症复发、转移，最终失去生命，由于当前主流医学对中医药治疗等方法的排斥，能够前来用生命修复治疗的癌症患者，往往在接受诊治时已经到了晚期，即使如此，我们仍然取得了良好的治疗效果。取得疗效的关键在于治疗原则不能因循守旧，医学理论必须有发展和创新，而不是将主流医学尚谈不上理想的治疗方法作为唯一的救命稻草。

　　我们已经陆续介绍了部分患者的案例并出版了几本书。本书在已出版图书的基础上，进一步用真实的病例介绍了晚期癌症患者使用生命修复的中医药治疗而致生命之树常青的事实。书中为保护患者隐私，没有公开姓名。所有关于患者病情、病程、疾病的严重程度、患病时间、检查报告等所有资料都是真实可查的。目前所有患者都恢复了正常的生活，从事着不同的工作。

关于所使用的药物，我们在前面几本书中都有所介绍，在本书中也列出了主要治疗原则和常用中药。这些患者朋友在长期的生活和工作中，病情和身体状态都会有变化，不可能只是使用一两个现成的药方，每个病例经年累月的诊疗记录只能是记录在病历上，无法在书中全部展现，所以我们只能尽可能列出最常用的治疗原则和常用中药。那些一剂方药包治百病的说法是毫无根据的。

我们已对所治疗的各种不同晚期癌症的万余病例进行了医学统计学处理和总结。结果显示，生命修复中医药治疗方法的治疗效果明确，并有显著性差异。

本书的另一个重要内容是较为详细地介绍了当前急需了解认识的防癌抗癌知识。这些内容可能与某些以前的认识或是以营利为目的宣传不相符合，但却是实际存在并随着社会的发展不断出现的有损健康、容易导致疾病的各种因素。防癌抗癌是全社会应当关注的重要问题，我们需要为维护公众和个人的健康而共同努力。

最后，希望患者朋友抛弃担忧和压力，鼓起勇气，充满信心，把握时机，正确治疗，与癌抗争，最终战胜癌症。也希望大家共同关心防癌抗癌的各个方面，提高健康水平和抗癌成效。

我也借此机会，衷心感谢那些支持我们工作的朋友。中医药学博大精深，源远流长，希望我们能够继续将它发扬光大，为患者和社会贡献一份微薄之力。

吴　锦

E-mail：liferepair@126.com

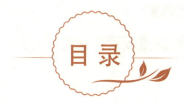

目 录

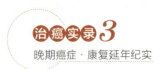

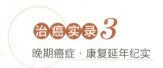

癌症治疗的历史和现状

根据世界卫生组织（WHO）2018 年最新报道，全球癌症发病率和死亡率仍呈迅速上升趋势。世界卫生组织公布的数据表明，全球每年约有 880 万人死于癌症，占全球每年死亡总人数近六分之一。每年有 1400 多万宗新发癌症病例，预计到 2030 年，这一数字将增加到 2100 多万宗。

可以看出，在全世界抗癌大军的努力下，癌症治疗取得了一定的进展和成绩，但是远远达不到"成功""满意"的程度。当前抗癌新药如雨后春笋一般不断涌现，各种广告铺天盖地，很难说这其中没有利欲的驱使。

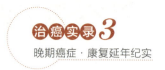
◇ **手术切除**

　　早期西医的治癌方法只是手术切除癌病灶，叫做手术根治，认为只要癌瘤没有了，癌就没有了。于是，人们以为手术能够根除癌症，就急不可待地做手术。然而，患癌的原因并没有因手术的切除而消失，贸然进行的手术反而大大破坏了器官组织功能和结构，于是癌肿很快复发、转移。时至今日，只要能够手术及再次手术的患者，仍然一而再、再而三地进行手术，这使得患者的生命力不断被消耗，并加速了癌瘤的转移最终促成了患者的死亡。

◇ **化学药物治疗**

　　在单纯以手术等方法治疗癌症出现无数次的失败之后，人们意识到了这些方法是不能治愈癌症的。最典型而且一直在作为指导肿瘤治疗的主要理论就是最著名的"杀死癌细胞"理论。100年前，西方科学家发现和发明了抗生素杀死细菌，拯救了大量因为细菌感染而生病的患者。之后开始采用抗生素杀灭细菌的方法治疗癌症，即使用大量具有强烈杀伤性的化学药物，旨在消灭所有癌细胞，"杀死最后一个癌细胞"。但是，这样的治疗方法并没有像抗生素杀菌那样奏效。因为癌细胞不像细菌那样是由外界入侵人体的外来物。各式各样的化疗药物都是在"杀死癌细胞"这个著名理论的指导下产生的。这就是化疗。

◇ 放射治疗

化疗没有取得意料之中的成功，治癌的队伍中又加上了使用放射线杀癌细胞的方法。从手术治癌到化疗治癌再到放疗（电疗）治癌，这些治疗方法在美国及全球前后用了 70 多年时间，效果到底如何？应该并不理想，且不良反应不少。有人作了调查，这 70 年，医生将手术、化疗和放疗作为治疗癌症的必用方法，已施用于数以亿计的患者身上。

◇ 靶向治疗

80 年代，癌症病因学说又有了新的理论，即癌症是患者细胞基因变异导致的，并找到了某些部位的癌基因，随之更为新潮的理论不断出现。在这些新理论的指导下，抗癌新药层出不穷，给它们的生产者带来了巨大利润。

◇ 免疫疗法

继靶向治疗的浪潮之后，免疫疗法闪亮登场。

然而，日本癌症专家近藤诚指出："癌症看上去像是与人的免疫能力有关，似乎是由于人体的免疫能力低下造成的，于是越来越多的人开始把目光转移到免疫疗法上去。免疫系统在人

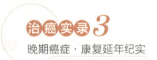

体被细菌、病毒、毒素等外来物质入侵时，的确会产生很大的作用，因为淋巴细胞能够分辨出这些成分到底来自自身还是外部。但当临床上已经检查出癌细胞时，就是证明淋巴细胞已经无法识别并阻止癌细胞了。淋巴细胞识别外敌的能力在诞生时就已被定型，后期无法更改，因此不管在后期怎么提高，也不可能被强化，所以说免疫疗法是没有意义的。"

19 年前晚期肺癌，如今庆贺 80 大寿

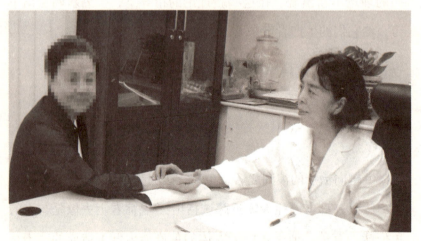

🎧 2018 年 7 月解太太来研究中心时留影

解太太于 1999 年专程去美国做了肺癌手术，手术切除了左上肺叶及左下肺叶的两个肿瘤。手术后她从美国返回香港，认为美国的医疗水平先进，她应该不会再有问题了。

但是好景不长，两年多后，解太太常有胸闷气促，咳嗽多痰，她感到与手术之前的症状很相似，于是又去医院进行检查，经磁共振及 CT 扫描检查，发现双肺均有新的肿瘤出现，两肺共有四个新的肿瘤，脑部也有一阴影。

解太太经多方咨询，了解到这种情况很不乐观，主刀医生对她的病况很了解，他认为虽然有先进的医疗技术，但这种术后肿瘤复发的病况是很严重的，目前实际上也没有有效的治疗方法，即使再次手术，医生心中也并无把握。

解太太只好试探问问，用中医药治疗可以吗？医生虽然并不了解中医药，但在没有更好办法的情况下，中医药作为一种新的方法进行尝试未尝不可，所以赞同她试用中医药治疗。于是解太太来寻求生命修复中医药治疗，开始服用中药。

当时她全身疲累无力，精神差、失眠、气促、胸闷、呼吸不能连续，每说一句话即需要大力换一口气。

治疗原则

健中培元，祛邪攻癌。

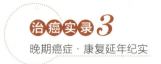

治疗方案

(1) 常用中药：熟地黄、山药、百合、蛤蚧、半夏、杏仁、苏子、牡蛎、炙甘草、麦冬、肉苁蓉、重楼等。

(2) 消瘤丸同时服用。

经过生命修复中医药治疗，解太太的症状逐渐缓解，她自己也感觉在慢慢恢复。半年左右再做检查，四个新的病灶全部消失。自解太太患肺癌至今，寒来暑往，已有十九个年头。她每年做检查，结果都显示肺癌没有再复发。她再没有使用过任何化疗、放射治疗、靶向治疗等治疗方法。

今年初，解太太喜迎八十岁寿辰，全家为庆贺她绝路逢生十九年，特择宴席，各方嘉宾云集，非常喜庆。

肺癌是恶性肿瘤中发病率高、恶性程度高、死亡率高的癌症。除化疗之外，尽管各种靶向治疗、免疫治疗层出不穷，肺癌仍是最恶性和最常见的癌症。解太太虽然经过了手术切除原发癌症病灶，但是二年之后在没有手术的另一侧肺部发现了三个转移病灶，脑部也出现了病灶。这种情况在肺癌患者中是很常见的。如按照常规治疗，并不能期望会有很好的结果。用生命修复中医药治疗，解太太已经平安愉快地度过了十九个春秋。

附：患者相关检查报告

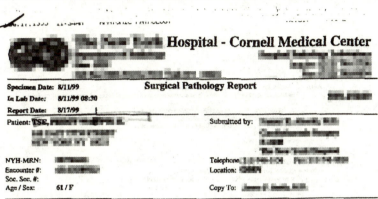

Hospital - Cornell Medical Center

Surgical Pathology Report

Specimen Date: 8/11/99

In Lab Date: 8/11/99 08:30

Report Date: 8/17/99

Patient: TSE,

NYH-MRN:

Encounter #:

Soc. Sec. #:

Age / Sex: 61 / F

Submitted by:

Telephone

Location:

Copy To:

CLINICAL INFORMATION:

61 year-old woman undergoing a left thoracotomy.

Specimen submitted: A. Wedge biopsy left lower lobe; B. Wedge biopsy left lower lobe; C. Portion of left sixth rib; D. Left upper lobe; E. Level 7 node.

INTRAOPERATIVE DIAGNOSIS:

A. Frozen section diagnosis: Adenocarcinoma.

B. Frozen section diagnosis: Adenocarcinoma.

GROSS DESCRIPTION:

A. Received fresh in the frozen lab labeled with the patient's name, unit number and "wedge biopsy left lower lobe" is a 2.5 x 2.0 x 1.0 cm. wedge biopsy with a 2.5 cm. stapled edge. The pleural surface is unremarkable and sectioning reveals a 1.0 x 1.0 x 0.8 cm. tan semifirm nodule; one half is frozen as AFS. The remainder of the nodule and lung parenchyma are submitted in AFSC through A9.

B. Received fresh in the frozen section lab labeled with the patient's name, unit number and "wedge biopsy left lower lobe" is a 2.0 x 1.0 x 0.8 cm. lung wedge biopsy with a 2.0 cm. long stapled edge. The pleura is unremarkable and sectioning reveals a 0.5 cm. poorly circumscribed tan semifirm area frozen entirely as BFS and resubmitted in BPSC. Remaining lung parenchyma is submitted in B1 through B4.

C. Received fresh and labeled with the patient's name, unit number, and "portion of left sixth rib" are several fragments of skeletal muscle and rib measuring in aggregate 1.2 x 0.8 x 0.4 cm. The specimen is decalcified and submitted entirely in C1.

D. Received fresh and labeled with the patient's name, unit number, and "left upper lobe" is a 15 x 9.0 x 4.0 cm. left upper lobectomy specimen with a 9.5 cm. serpiginous stapled edge around the hilum. The pleural surface is remarkable only for a 2.0 cm. gray pearly fibrous area at the apex. The unremarkable bronchovascular resection margin measures 2.0 x 1.0 cm. and numerous soft tan-black peribronchial lymph nodes measure from 0.2 to 0.4 cm. The specimen is sectioned to reveal 1.5 x 1.5 x 1.4 cm. poorly circumscribed stellate tan-gray firm mass in the basal-lateral portion of the lobe coming within 0.2 cm. of overlying pleura, 1.0 cm. of the medial stapled resection margin and 3.0 cm. of the bronchovascular resection margins. Adjacent and remaining lung parenchyma is remarkable only for prominent vessels and slightly enlarged air spaces. The specimen is photographed. Summary of sections: D1-bronchovascular resection margin; D2 through D4-tumor in relation to overlying pleura; D5 through D9-lung parenchyma, representative sections; D10-peribronchial lymph nodes.

E. Received fresh labeled with the patient's name, unit number and "level 7 node" is a 1.2 x 0.5 x 0.3 cm. aggregate of soft tan-black tissue submitted entirely in E1. (DF)

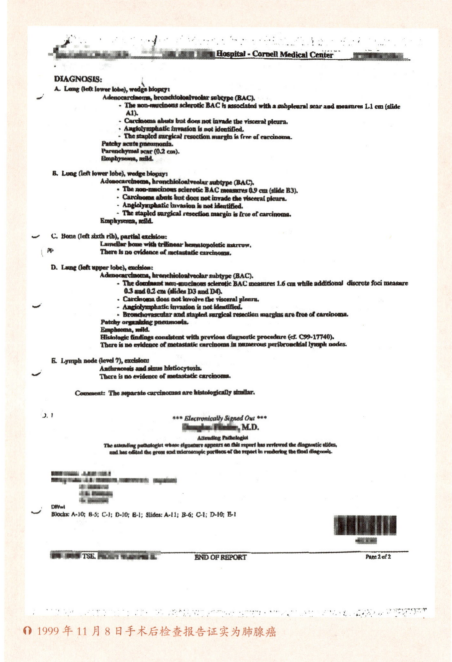

Hospital - Cornell Medical Center

DIAGNOSIS:

A. Lung (left lower lobe), wedge biopsy:
Adenocarcinoma, bronchioloalveolar subtype (BAC).
- The non-mucinous sclerotic BAC is associated with a subpleural scar and measures 1.1 cm (slide A1).
- Carcinoma abuts but does not invade the visceral pleura.
- Angiolymphatic invasion is not identified.
- The stapled surgical resection margin is free of carcinoma.
Patchy acute pneumonia.
Parenchymal scar (0.2 cm).
Emphysema, mild.

B. Lung (left lower lobe), wedge biopsy:
Adenocarcinoma, bronchioloalveolar subtype (BAC).
- The non-mucinous sclerotic BAC measures 0.9 cm (slide B3).
- Carcinoma abuts but does not invade the visceral pleura.
- Angiolymphatic invasion is not identified.
- The stapled surgical resection margin is free of carcinoma.
Emphysema, mild.

C. Bone (left sixth rib), partial excision:
Lamellar bone with trilinear hematopoietic marrow.
There is no evidence of metastatic carcinoma.

D. Lung (left upper lobe), excision:
Adenocarcinoma, bronchioloalveolar subtype (BAC).
- The dominant non-mucinous sclerotic BAC measures 1.6 cm while additional discrete foci measure 0.3 and 0.2 cm (slides D3 and D4).
- Carcinoma does not involve the visceral pleura.
- Angiolymphatic invasion is not identified.
- Bronchovascular and stapled surgical resection margins are free of carcinoma.
Patchy organizing pneumonia.
Emphysema, mild.
Histologic findings consistent with previous diagnostic procedure (cf. C99-17740).
There is no evidence of metastatic carcinoma in numerous peribronchial lymph nodes.

E. Lymph node (level 7), excision:
Anthracosis and sinus histiocytosis.
There is no evidence of metastatic carcinoma.

Comment: The separate carcinomas are histologically similar.

*** Electronically Signed Out ***
M.D.
Attending Pathologist
The attending pathologist whose signature appears on this report has reviewed the diagnostic slides,
and has edited the gross and microscopic portions of the report in rendering the final diagnosis.

DP=i
Blocks: A-10; B-5; C-1; D-10; E-1; Slides: A-11; B-6; C-1; D-10; E-1

TSE.   END OF REPORT   Page 2 of 2

🎧 1999 年 11 月 8 日手术后检查报告证实为肺腺癌

████████HOSPITAL
SCANNING DEPARTMENT
(CT, MR, NM, Mammography, U/S, Bone Densitometry)

████████████████████████

Tel.: ████████████████████

REPORT FOR MRI/CT/NM SCANNING EXAMINATION

████ : CT ████████ 02   **EXAM. DATE** : Tue. 18 Jun. 2002
NAME : Wai

ID No. : B24████

AGE / SEX: 64 F
DATE : Tue. 18 Jun. 2002   **HOSPITAL** : OUT-PATIENT
EXAM. : CT of Thorax

CONTRAST MEDIUM : Iopamiro 370   **REF. DR.** : ████████████

CLINICAL HISTORY:

Bronchioalveolar cell carcinoma for follow-up. Small meningioma in brain, definite, not a metastasis also for follow-up.

RADIOLOGICAL REPORT:

5 mm collimation high resolution axial helical scans have been performed with and without contrast injection. One set of non-contrast images from the previous examination on 1 December, 2001 is also printed for comparison. A minute 2 mm nodule is shown in the anterior aspect of the right lower lung field is again shown (page 4, image 39). This lesion was present in previous examination also image 39. Previous opinion was said it is benign and this is a correct diagnosis. In the meantime the lesion has not increase in size at all.

There are total of four new lesions identifiable. One is located in the antero-medial aspect of the right lower lung about 2.5 cm above the level of the 2 mm lesion and shown in image 34. Its size is 26 x 19 mm along the transaxial plane. It is immediately subpleural in location and close to midline. Prior to contrast injection, density measurement ranging from 5 to 20. After contrast injection, there is enhancement ranging from 15 units to 40 units. A second lesion is shown in the shape of a fan and it is quite small in size measuring no more than 2 cm in diameter and is located in the posterior portion of the left lung base (image 47). It did not exist in previous examination. A third lesion is noted in the posterior right lung base. It is quite hazy in character and poorly defined in the boundaries. 1 mm images show the same characteristics. It may well be an area of pneumonitis and so is the second lesion. A fourth lesion is shown which is of the same hazy character and located in the postero-medial aspect of the left upper lung.

Post-contrast scan shows no sign of any mediastinal or hilar lymphadenopathy. Regional bones show no metastatic disease.

♪ 2002 年 6 月 18 日 MRI/CT/SCAN 报告双肺发现有 4 个新的病灶，它们分别位于：①右肺下叶；②左肺底；③右肺底；④左肺上叶

Hospital

Scanning Department
(CT, MR, NM, PET Scan, Bone Densitometry)

REPORT FOR MRI/CT/NM/PET SCANNING EXAMINATION

OUR REF. : CT ▮▮▮▮ 02   EXAM. DATE : Sat, 7 Dec, 2002
NAME : Wai
ID No. : B24
AGE / SEX : 64 F
DATE : Mon, 9 Dec, 2002   HOSPITAL : OUT-PATIENT
XAM. : CT of Thorax

CONTRAST MEDIUM : Iopamiro 370   REF. DR. : ▮▮▮▮▮▮▮▮▮

CLINICAL HISTORY:

Bronchio-alveolar cell tumour, treated, for sequential follow-up.

RADIOLOGICAL REPORT:

Helical scan has been performed with high resolution technique. Left upper lung field shows linear densities representing scars both in the peripheral lung and in the perihilar region. Comparison with previous examination indicates that all the shadows existing in the lungs were previously presented including the small nodule in the anterior aspect of the right lung base (image 44) which has not been enlarging at all with the passage of time. Post-contrast scan demonstrates that the different major areas of the mediastinum are also normal without enlarged lymph node while the regional bones including the thoracic spine show no sign of plastic or lytic lesion.

OPINION :

This post-treatment follow-up study is quite satisfactory. Last examination was done exactly 3 months ago in 7th Sept, 2002. No change is observed and there is no sign of any recurrence of tumour in the lungs, mediastinum, hilum, pleural space, regional bones or chest wall.

NO. OF FILMS : 0 14" x 17"   SIGNED

DR. ▮▮▮▮▮▮▮▮

⋂ 2002年12月7日 CT SCAN 报告与3个月前检查比较, 治疗反应良好, 在肺部、纵隔、肺门、胸膜、胸骨等部位均没有见到有任何肿瘤复发

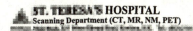

ST. TERESA'S HOSPITAL
Scanning Department (CT, MR, NM, PET)

Exam No. : **CT**

Patient Name : TSE		Chi. Name :	
ID No. :	Sex / Age : F / 80Yr	Visit No. :	
Ref. Dr. : Dr.		Bed No. :	Date : 13-04-2018
Exam : **CT - Thorax: Low Dose Screening**		Ref. From :	

Copy

PT - 4/13/18
CT - Thorax

IMAGING REPORT:

Clinical Information:

Remote history of alveolar cell carcinoma of lung (left side) treated in Sloan Kettering Cancer Center in New York. For long term follow-up.

Imaging Technique:

Non-contrast axial helical scan of the thorax with low dose technique was performed.

Imaging Findings:

Linear five calcified fibrotic scars are noted in the anterior aspect of the left apex. Tiny calcified granuloma is also shown in the posteromedial aspect of the right mid lung. Another non-calcified nodule is also shown in the medial aspect of the right mid lung. Major airway shows rather extensive wall calcifications and spotty calcifications are also found in the aortic arch. No other abnormal shadow is noted in both lung fields and the appearance of the lungs is about the same as in previous examination performed in November 2015.

Opinion:

No active disease is shown in the lungs. History of alveolar cell carcinoma treated back in the remote past is noted. There is no sign of malignant recurrence. Tiny non-calcified and calcified but non-active tuberculomas are shown in the lungs. No active disease of any kind is noted at this point in time.

No. of image prints : 4   No. of DVD : 1
Remark :
NGWH
Report No. :

on 14-04-2018 @ 15:20:30   Page 1 of 1

🔈 2018 年 4 月 13 日检查报告示无肿瘤复发转移

看看医学专家怎么说

　　日本抗癌专家近藤诚医生独创的乳房保留法至今仍是手术治疗乳腺癌的标准方法。同样，他也是大胆对抗"抗癌药联盟"的斗士，提出了惊世骇俗的西药抗癌药无效论。他的著作中有以下论述。

◇ 抗癌药的副作用不容忽视

除了手术之外，服用抗癌药物也可能置患者于死地。2002年，一种万众期待的肺癌抗癌药易瑞沙作为"梦幻新药"登场。但是服用过该药的患者因间质性肺炎而致死的事件频发，该药发售半年就已经让 200 人失去了生命，10 年来累计有超过 850人因这种药死去。更让人气愤的是，这种药始终没有体现出可以延长患者寿命的效果。

抗癌药有一定的细胞毒性，虽然在一定时期内能够缩小肿瘤，但总有一天肿瘤会再次长大，而那时候患者的身体早已被抗癌药猛烈的毒性侵蚀，从而会让患者更加痛苦，得不偿失。

◇ 手术切口处癌细胞最易复发

那么在没有癌症治疗方法的时代，患者的病情又是怎样发展的呢？我发现过这样一组观察数据，这些数据令人不禁深思。

那是 1803—1933 年间 250 名英国乳腺癌患者的观察记录。在 X 线机都没有的时代里，诊断癌症的依据是看肿块是否变大或者是否突破皮肤。从当时英国乳腺癌患者的数据中我发现患者 5 年生存率为 18%，10 年生存率为 6%。

进入 20 世纪以后，手术切除法诞生，世界从此进入了"把可疑疾病全部切掉"的时代。患者如果被诊断出患有乳腺癌，就会把乳房切到肋骨附近，连淋巴结也一并去掉，从那时候起，

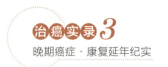

"霍尔斯特德手术"盛行了近70年。霍尔斯特德本人发表了420名乳腺癌患者的生存率，手术死亡率占4%，而5年生存率为18%，10年生存率为6%。

通过对比两份数据，我们可以发现不管切掉多少，或者什么都不做，患者的生存率都没有改变。在这一前提下，保留乳房的"乳房保留疗法"成为现今的主流。但"发现癌症以后尽早切除"的想法在医学界并没有那么容易被化解。

对于早发现的肿瘤，大部分人都是希望能在第一时间将其切除，但手术可能导致更为糟糕的后果，比如出现转移或者复发。

然而当今社会虽然比过去进步和发达了很多，世人还是像过去的人们那样故步自封，对癌症的真相视而不见。例如美国的最新调查发现因肺癌转移而使用抗癌药进行治疗的患者将近七成，约八成大肠癌患者都相信"抗癌药能治愈癌症"。

其实不管是哪个国家的医生、制药公司都希望患者尽可能地长时间接受治疗，使用他们的昂贵药物，所以他们把"在某些时候抗癌药虽能使肿瘤缩小，但不能够治愈"这样的事实隐瞒了起来。

◇ **开腹手术可能会让癌细胞转移至腹膜**

对待癌症晚期患者的手术治疗要无比谨慎，因为手术部位是癌细胞最容易滋生的地方，非常容易引起癌症的复发。

开腹手术还特别容易引起患者体内癌细胞进行腹膜转移。

本来人体内的腹膜是非常光滑的，很难被依附，而且癌细胞也无法轻易进入到里面。但是一旦在腹膜处动手术的话，切口处会变得十分粗糙，这样使得癌细胞能轻易依附在上面并增殖。结果导致正常细胞的保护屏障崩溃，癌细胞泛滥。这种情况又类似播种，因此癌细胞落到腹腔内又被称为"腹膜播种"。腹膜转移是相当麻烦和难以控制的一种癌细胞转移症状，如大肠癌、胃癌等需要在腹部进行开刀手术的则会使这种风险有增无减，因此，对于这两类癌症，一定要仔细考虑后再作选择。对于胃癌切除手术，欧美国家已经普遍不再将淋巴结一并切除，因为切与不切都不会对患者的生存率有所改变。

◇ 抗癌药本身具有一定的细胞毒性

所有的抗癌药都具有一定的细胞毒性，它在杀死癌细胞的同时也杀死正常细胞。因为正常细胞比癌细胞分裂得更快，所以大量正常细胞都会被抗癌药杀掉，从而导致患者很快死去。

另一方面，即使抗癌药能把99%普通癌细胞消灭掉，但顽强的癌干细胞存活下来的可能性非常大，一旦癌干细胞幸存下来，它们很快就会进行转移、增殖，卷土重来。

我以前在美国留学的时候脑子里想的都是希望尽快学会欧美国家关于癌症的所有先进治疗方法，后来却发现很多患者因抗癌药的毒性而饱受折磨，而且有不少人明显更早地结束了生命。

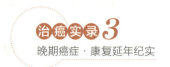
这让我十分困惑，开始怀疑抗癌药"治疗效果"的数据有虚假成分，为了知道抗癌药真正的治疗效果到底是怎么样的，我决定把世界上有临床数据的抗癌药治疗相关论文从头看起分析甚至追溯到癌症的本质、性质，在理解这些的基础上再去思考治疗的效果。

结果从数据中我发现很多抗癌药的试验都有制药公司成员的参与，他们公司的名字被堂堂正正地写进了论文。

◇ 抗癌药是把双刃剑

最近有很多效果很好的抗癌药，"这些药物疗效都不错"。这是医生们与患者交谈中常出现的一句话，然而患者却不知道很多"梦幻新药"都曾引起过可怕的死亡事件。我在前面也已经说过了，最典型的例子是 2002 年面世的新型肺癌抗癌药——易瑞沙（Iressa，通用名：吉非替尼），当时该药曾号称"几乎没有副作用"，结果发售不久就相继出现患者因副作用致死的情况。

正常情况下抗癌药会把癌细胞和正常细胞一并杀死，导致患者出现呕吐、腹泻、掉发等严重的副作用。易瑞沙当时也曾被这样评价过："对所有癌细胞和某些分子会产生作用，狙击癌细胞的能力极其优秀。"

据统计，易瑞沙发售于 2002 年 7 月，至当年 12 月为止就有 358 人出现间质性肺炎，其中死亡 114 人。而日本国立癌症研究中心中央医院使用易瑞沙的 112 名患者中死亡 4 人。东北大学在 60 天内有 18 人使用了易瑞沙，其中 4 人出现严重的间质性肺炎，2 人死亡。

另外，多个临床试验数据结果表明"没有服用易瑞沙的人活得更久"，如今易瑞沙已被视为"没有延长寿命效果"的药物。

无数的患者被没有延长寿命效果的抗癌药所欺骗，盲目相信所谓的"划时代新药""几乎没有副作用"这些话，结果导致自己挣扎于痛苦之中，最后在痛苦中死去。

我一直坚信不管是抗癌药还是靶向治疗药物都是有一定毒性的，而事实也是如此，很多患者一旦开始使用抗癌药，体质就会急剧下降、病情恶化并易感染，直至最后死亡。所以使用抗癌药是在用生命做赌注，进行一次没有胜算的赌博。

◇ 免疫疗法的治疗真相

由于癌症看上去像是与人的免疫能力密切相关，似乎是由于人体的免疫能力低下造成的，于是越来越多的人开始把目光转移到免疫疗法上去。那事实上又是如何呢？

其实过去也曾经出现不少相关研究。研究者把采集到的淋巴细胞样本放到试管中培养，等淋巴细胞的能力被强化以后再放回人体中。后来证实这种做法只对一部分恶性黑色素瘤有效，而且只是缩小了肿瘤而已，对其他癌症几乎不起作用，所以研究者们的热情很快就消退了。

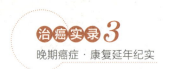

◇ 三大疗法可能导致癌症的扩散和复发

中国的肿瘤专家院士汤剑猷教授研究癌症一辈子，在各个场合的演讲中，都告诫癌症患者不要轻易开刀。那些抱有一刀下去就能解决问题的态度未必正确。

长久以来，西医以手术、化疗、放疗为主的治癌方法一直被奉为最正统、最科学的治疗方法。但是，随着时间的推移，越来越多统计数字的出现，使人们逐渐认识到这些方法对癌症的治疗效果是不好的，还需要在其他领域中寻找治疗之路。虽然西方没有中医药学，但越来越多的西医在发掘具有抗癌功效的天然植物，日本就有以中医药学为基础发展的汉方医学。中医药学经过几千年的发展，对天然药物的性味、归经、用法和功效等的掌握有着无可比拟的优越之处，较之这些年西方才找出来的一些植物来说，我们有更充足的经验来发展中医药抗癌理论。

日本医学界的许多专家近年来也开始逐步使用天然疗法，摆脱常规西医治疗的羁绊。济阳医师是专治消化器官的外科医师，行医超过四十年，更是日本抗癌饮食研究首屈一指的名医。身为外科医生的他，原本以为医疗的最大贡献必然在于手术与开刀技术的精准——精确地切除患者的病灶，再配合化学疗法或放射治疗。但经过对手术患者的追踪调查，他发现即使手术再成功，患者的 5 年生存率仍仅有 52%。这样的结果让他大感惊讶并自责："难道不能再想想办法？"在反复思索后，他开始寻求自然疗法，以新鲜蔬果汁饮食为主进行辅助治疗，取得了比单用西医治疗更好的疗效。

台湾抗癌医师黄鼎殷指出，过去 100 年来随着医学的不断进步，癌症的治疗出现了两种情况：一是癌症患者的存活年数及生活品质并没有太大改善；二是患癌人数不减反增。

现代医学的癌症治疗通常只有三条路可走：手术、化疗与放射线治疗。

手术治疗的对象除了病灶与肿瘤之外，还包括在手术过程中宁可多切除也不放过的组织或器官，如淋巴结就会被取出以供分析是否发生癌细胞转移，同时合并采用的化疗或放射治疗也是用来在手术前先根除所有转移中或已形成的癌细胞。

化学疗法，大家都知道它会造成细胞免疫力降低，如白细胞或是淋巴球（亦称为"白细胞数"）的功能不足，此外，还会造成恶心、呕吐、脱发、精神不济、疲倦与体质下降等副作用，甚至引起败血症或多重器官衰竭，进而使患者无力对抗致命的细菌感染，让患者产生很多的不适。

放射治疗也会造成组织坏死、纤维化及接受放射线的局部区域循环不良等副作用，治疗之后可能会出现严重不适及部分器官失能，如淋巴肿瘤就是个好例子。虽然近年来已经出现更先进的放射线疗法，可以利用立体造影机器定位肿瘤，并从不同角度施以不同的放射线来达到杀死癌肿瘤的目的，但是仍会有副作用的产生。

这些疗法都只是局部性的治疗，缺乏整体性的观念，并不是每一个癌症患者都能完整地表达他们的感觉，不论是哪一种疗法，癌症患者都不被当作一个正常人来尊重，反而像是被作为不需被疼惜的对象对待。现代医学的肿瘤科医师在养成教育

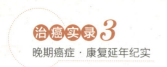
中也都会被训练成治疗患者时应当不带感情地保持中立。

　　假设你罹患癌症，情况很可能是你的医生会很快地建议你说，可行的疗法"唯有手术、化疗和（或）放疗"。

　　假设你长了肿瘤，医生便会试图靠手术切除它。在切除肿瘤后，他们通常会建议用含毒性的毒药做化学疗法，以杀死任何可能残存的癌细胞，最后以放射线疗法为尾声，烧死所有残余的癌细胞。这就是为什么我及其他许多人会把三大疗法形容成砍、毒、烧的原因。就是这种有毒的疗法误导我们相信，那是治疗癌症的最佳疗法。

　　而导致癌症的扩散和复发的，也正是这三大疗法。

　　手术往往是造成癌症扩散的原因，医生微小的失误便可能使数百万个癌细胞慢慢渗入患者的血液中。化学疗法是有毒的，会致癌，摧毁红细胞，使免疫系统瘫痪，并破坏维系生命的重要器官。艾伦·李文博士说过："这个国家（美国）的癌症患者大部分都死于化学疗法。化学疗法无法消灭乳癌、结肠癌或肺癌，这一事实已被证实多年，但医生们仍在使用化疗对付这些癌症。"没错，三大疗法已在许多案例中被证明会缩短寿命。

◇　肿瘤缩小 ≠ 延长寿命

　　Dr. Ralph Moss 说：必须提一下，化疗药物刚开始是源于第一及第二次世界大战中的生物武器"芥气"实验。暴露在芥气中会导致快速生长组织的毁灭，所以就有人推测，既然癌症生长得很迅速，这些毒素应该也可以杀死癌组织。这个嘛，他们是对的……暴露在这些气体中的确可以杀死癌组织。化疗和放疗真的可以缩小肿瘤的大小并且杀死癌细胞，但是，肿瘤缩小就等于治疗癌症了吗？这两者之间有直接的相关性吗？答案是"不"。

Dr. Ralph Moss 还说："假如你能将肿瘤缩小 50% 以上达 28 天，你就达到食品药物管理局对有效药物所制定的标准，这叫作回应率，所以你得到了回应……（但是）当你检视接受这种治疗对寿命是否有任何的延长作用时，你所看到的是各式各样的幻术、庆祝摆脱病魔纠缠的载歌载舞等。但到最后还是没能证明化疗在绝大多数案例中真的能够延长寿命，他们还制造了关于化疗的天大谎言：在缩小肿瘤大小和延长患者寿命之间有相关性。"以下才是我们应当了解的真相。1942 年，史隆凯特琳癌症纪念中心默默地开始用那些芥气衍生物治疗乳癌，结果没有人被治愈。1943 年左右耶鲁也展开了化疗试验，治疗 160 位患者，同样也没有人被治愈。但是，既然化疗能够缩小肿瘤，研究人员便很兴奋地宣布化疗试验是"成功的"。我认为我们需要精确定义"成功"的意义，不是吗？

解剖研究已证明，实际上癌症患者在癌症有机会杀死他们之前，就先死于常规疗法。

如果化疗药物缩减了肿瘤的大小，那么该药物必定是有效的。不过，有效的意义究竟是什么？表示患者会活得更久吗？不，有确切的文件记录指出，肿瘤缩小和较长的癌症存活率之间是没什么关系的。

晚期鼻咽癌多发骨转移，奋斗事业 12 年

方先生 30 多岁，在一家公司当经理，每日忙忙碌碌。半年多来，他经常有头痛、耳鸣、鼻塞、眼痛、视物模糊、眩晕等症状。开始以为是工作太忙，经常熬夜的缘故，过段时间就会没事。但没多久病情加重，视物模糊，耳鸣如潮，头痛剧烈，不得已去医院看医生，结果没那么简单，医生让他做了不少检查，包括活组织检查，确诊为鼻咽癌晚期。

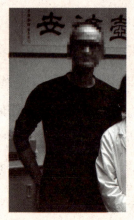

2018 年 6 月方先生在研究中心与医生留影

医院安排他做放疗，并告知：他的病情已属晚期，有广泛的骨转移，如各鼻窦、筛骨、蝶骨、颅骨、颈椎等都已有大范围的转移，而且肿瘤已侵犯视神经，即使做了放疗，肿瘤复发，继续转移及失明的可能性很大。他感到压力很大，经过一番考虑后，决定求助于生命修复治癌，一边放疗，一边前来吃中药。放疗之后，仍坚持不懈地中药治疗。

解毒化郁，散结消瘤。

治疗方案

(1) 常用中药：柴胡、黄芩、鱼腥草、山慈菇、八月札、浙贝母、鱼脑石、半夏、僵蚕、海浮石等。

(2) 消瘤丸同时服用。

中药以养阴清肺、化痰祛邪为主，可以有效地缓解放疗的副作用，如口干、失眠、耳鸣、不能进食等。更可喜的是，严重的肿瘤转移全部消失。如今已过去 12 年了，仍没有复发和转移，当时西医所说的 1 ~ 2 年之后会复发、转移并未发生，他完全战胜了癌症。

随着医疗水平的提高，鼻咽癌的治疗手段较过去已有明显改善，尤其是放射治疗，对癌细胞有直接的杀灭作用。但是副作用较大，损伤较大。对于晚期鼻咽癌治疗现状仍不理想，患者接受放射治疗之后，中医药学的观点一般认为有火热毒邪入侵，导致热毒过盛，化火灼津，患者会有口干、咽喉干燥疼痛、吞咽困难等阴虚内热及严重的放射性损伤症状，更为重要的是其他地方的转移病灶仍需大力治疗和控制，才能防止癌症卷土重来。在这种情况下，生命修复的中医药治疗发挥了很好的养阴、攻毒、抗癌作用，使患者能完全康复。

附：患者相关检查报告

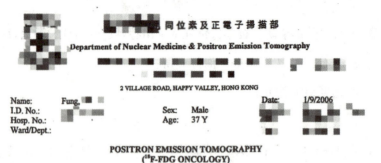

同位素及正電子掃描部

Department of Nuclear Medicine & Positron Emission Tomography

2 VILLAGE ROAD, HAPPY VALLEY, HONG KONG

Name: Fung, Date: 1/9/2006
I.D. No.: Sex: Male
Hosp. No.: Age: 37 Y
Ward/Dept.:

POSITRON EMISSION TOMOGRAPHY
(^{18}F-FDG ONCOLOGY)

History:

A 37 year-old gentleman presented with left epistaxis. Biopsy on 23/8/2006 confirmed nasopharyngeal carcinoma. Clinical and MRI showed disease in left nasal cavity extending up to the inferior aspect of ethmoidal-sphenoid junction medial to left bony orbit, left NP sidewall, roof of nasopharynx and neck is clear. PET scan is now performed for staging. Body weight, appetite and sleep are normal. Bowel movement and urination normal. No bone pain, no cough, no night sweat. Non-smoker, non-drinker. No history of hepatitis or tuberculosis. Did not take any herbs. Took boiled lingzhi for a few years for ~10 times a few years ago. No family history of TB and cancer.

Procedures:

Fasting blood glucose at 10:40 was 5.7 mmol/l. 60 mg Spasmonal was given p.o. 15 min before ^{18}FDG. 12.8 mCi of ^{18}F-FDG was injected at 10:50. PET-CT scan from base of skull to groin was performed at 11:52 (62 minutes after injection).

Findings:

SUVmax = Standardized Uptake Value Maximum
SUVavg = Standardized Uptake Value Average

Liver tissue normal reference uptake has a SUVmax of 2.86 and a SUVavg of 2.33. Delayed PET-CT SUVmax 2.11 and SUVavg 2.01.

A hypermetabolic mass can be seen in the anterior nasopharyngeal roof. This is consistent with clinical diagnosis of nasopharyngeal carcinoma(3.6 cm W x 3.1 cm H x 4.9 cm D, SUVmax 11.76, delayed SUVmax 12.99). The tumor anteriorly extends into the left posterior nasal choana and cephalically it protrudes cephalically into the inferior part of ethmoid sinus. Laterally it is situated proximal to the left supra-orbital fissure. There is no definite bony erosion can be identified. Inferiorly the tumor is at the level of upper border of C1 ring, and anteriorly in the nasal choana is just cephalic to the left nasal inferior concha. No definite hypermetabolic lymph node can be seen. There is some mild asymmetric with a mild increase on the

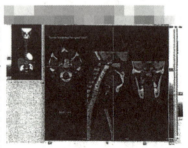

left side of the left jugulo-digastric node just posterior medial to the angle of left mandible. There is some tiny lymph node seen there more than the contralateral side.

Both lungs appear clear and the mediastinum shows normal physiological activities. The cardiac muscle shows normal increased uptake. The liver shows uniform uptake without any focal area of

同位素及正電子掃描部

Department of Nuclear Medicine & Positron Emission Tomography

hypermetabolism. The adrenal glands appear normal. There is no abnormal abdominal para-aortic lymph node. The bowel shows some physiological activity in the muscle of the intestine. There is no abnormal pelvic uptake. Both groins appear normal with no abnormal lymphadenopathy. There is no abnormal uptake in the prostate area.

<u>Impression:</u>

1. The findings are consistent with the clinical diagnosis of nasopharyngeal carcinoma situating in the nasopharyngeal roof area. The tumor anteriorly extends into the left posterior nasal choana and also cephalic protruding into the left ethmoid sinus. Laterally, the tumor is in close proximity to the optic nerve in the superior orbital fissure. There is no definite osseous erosion. The inferior border of the tumor would be about the plane of C1.

2. No macroscopic metastatic lymph node can be seen but some tiny lymph nodes in the left jugulo-digastric node show mild asymmetrical activity increased on the left side. Thus microscopic metastasis to the left jugulo-digastric nodes posterior medial to the angle of mandible cannot be completely excluded.

3. No distant metastasis can be seen.

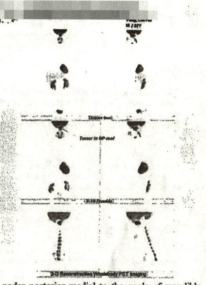

Thank you very much, Dr. Tsang, for your referral.

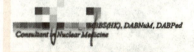

MBBS(HK), DABNuM, DABPed
Consultant in Nuclear Medicine

🎧 2006 年 9 月 1 日 CT 检查报告证实鼻咽癌，并有较广泛的颅骨及周围骨转移，已接近侵犯视神经

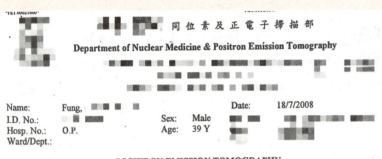

同位素及正電子掃描部

Department of Nuclear Medicine & Positron Emission Tomography

Name: Fung,

I.D. No.:

Hosp. No.: O.P.

Ward/Dept.:

Date: 18/7/2008

Sex: Male

Age: 39 Y

POSITRON EMISSION TOMOGRAPHY
(^{18}F-FDG ONCOLOGY)

<u>History</u>:

A 39 year-old gentleman with nasopharyngeal carcinoma diagnosed in 2006, status post chemoradiation therapy completed in 11/2006 for follow-up evaluation. He has been clinically asymptomatic.

<u>Radiopharmaceutical</u>: 11.3 mCi F-18 Fluorodeoxyglucose (^{18}FDG) injected intravenously.

<u>Findings</u>:

Limited whole body CT transmission and PET emission imaging began at 76 minutes after radiopharmaceutical administration (blood glucose 5.4 mmol/l), spanning a region from base of skull to upper thigh. 60 mg Spasmonal was given p.o. 15 min before ^{18}FDG administration.

Liver tissue normal reference uptake has a SUVmax of 2.95.

Comparison is made with prior PET scan dated 24/1/2008.

There is mild decreased ^{18}FDG activity in the left side of the nasopharynx, unchanged since the prior study and consistent with post-treatment changes. There are no ^{18}FDG-avid or enlarged lymph nodes in bilateral neck and axillae.

Bilateral lung fields are clear with no pulmonary nodules. There are no hypermetabolic or enlarged lymph nodes in the mediastinum.

There is normal diffuse ^{18}FDG activity in the liver and spleen. There are no hypermetabolic or enlarged lymph nodes in the celiac axis, retroperitoneal space of the abdomen and pelvis, and bilateral inguinal regions. There are no abnormal focal uptake in the pancreas and the GI tract. The adrenals are normal in size and non-^{18}FDG-avid.

The rest of the visualized structures show normal radiotracer activity. There are no abnormal focal uptake in the bony structures to suggest osseous metastasis.

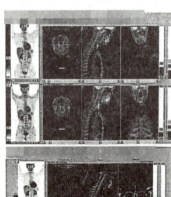

同位素及正電子掃描部

Department of Nuclear Medicine & Positron Emission Tomography

Impression:

1. Negative PET scan showing no evidence of local tumor recurrence.
2. There is no evidence of lymph node or distant metastasis.

Thank you very much, █████, for your referral.

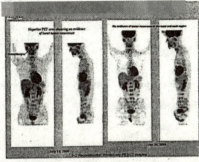

M.B.,B.S.(H.K.), A.B.I.M., A.B.N.M., F.R.C.R.(U.K.), F.H.K.C.R., F.H.K.A.M.(Radiology)
Department of Nuclear Medicine & P.E.T. █████

🎧 2008 年 7 月 18 日检查报告证实肿瘤消失无复发

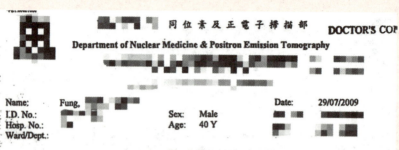

同位素及正電子掃描部
Department of Nuclear Medicine & Positron Emission Tomography
DOCTOR'S COP

Name: Fung,
I.D. No.:
Hosp. No.:
Ward/Dept.:

Sex: Male
Age: 40 Y

Date: 29/07/2009

POSITRON EMISSION TOMOGRAPHY
(^{18}F-FDG ONCOLOGY)

History:

40 year-old gentleman with nasopharyngeal carcinoma diagnosed in 2006, status post chemoradiation therapy completed in 11/2006, for follow-up evaluation. He has been clinically asymptomatic.

Radiopharmaceutical: 12.4 mCi F-18 Fluorodeoxyglucose (^{18}FDG) injected intravenously.

Findings:

Limited whole body CT transmission and PET emission imaging began at 59 minutes after radiopharmaceutical administration (blood glucose 5.5 mmol/l), spanning a region from base of skull to upper thigh. 60 mg Spasmonal was given p.o. 15 min before ^{18}FDG administration.

Liver tissue normal reference uptake has a SUVmax of 2.36.

Comparison is made with prior PET scan dated 18/07/2008.

There is no abnormal focal ^{18}FDG activity in the nasopharynx. There are no ^{18}FDG-avid or enlarged lymph nodes in bilateral neck and axillae. There is mild asymmetric increased ^{18}FDG activity in the left base of tongue that is within normal physiologic variation. This was also seen in PET scans of 01/2008 and 07/2008 and has been stable.

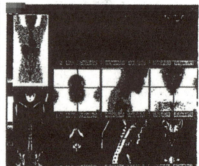

Bilateral lung fields are clear with no pulmonary nodules. There are no hypermetabolic or enlarged lymph nodes in the mediastinum and bilateral hilar regions.

In the abdomen, there is normal diffuse ^{18}FDG activity in the liver and spleen. There are no hypermetabolic lymph nodes in the celiac axis, retroperitoneal space of the abdomen and pelvis. There are no abnormal focal ^{18}FDG activities in the pancreas, kidneys and the GI tract. Adrenals are normal.

The rest of the visualized structures show normal radiotracer activity. There are no hypermetabolic bone lesions to suggest osseous metastasis.

同位素及正電子掃描部

Department of Nuclear Medicine & Positron Emission Tomography

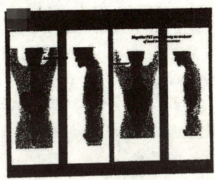

Impression:

1. Negative PET scan showing no evidence of local tumor recurrence.
2. There is no evidence of lymph node or distant metastasis.

Thank you very much, ███ for your referral.

M.B.B.S.(H.K.), A.B.I.M., A.B.N.M., F.R.C.R.(U.K.), F.H.K.C.R.,
F.H.K.A.M.(Radiology)
Department of Nuclear Medicine & P.E.T., ███

🎧 2009 年 7 月 29 日再次检查报告证实肿瘤全部消失无复发

中医治癌

◇ 癌症之名古籍已载

中医对癌瘤的认识源远流长。公元前 16 世纪至公元前 11 世纪殷商甲骨文即有"瘤"字出现，而《灵枢·刺节真邪论》也论述了"瘤"的分类。在《黄帝内经》中，"伏梁""癥积""肠覃""昔瘤""石瘕""石痈""乳岩"等都是有关瘤的记载。宋代的《卫济宝书》则有"癌"的论述，其音与"岩"同。"岩"的甲骨文是一个会意字，就是在山形之上，另加三个口形之石，表示巨石突起的山峰，其形即与癌字相似。小篆的"岩"是一个从山从严的形声字，用于描述疾病，表示肿瘤的凸凹与肿物的坚突。刘完素在《素问玄机原病式》中谓："夫水数一，道近而善；火数二，道远而恶。"其所列举的火热病证中就有"瘤气"。瘤气即具内浊积结、动乱参差之恶性。

在中医学古典文献《内经》中就有许多关于"瘤"的论述，如《灵枢·九针论》说："四时八风之客于经络之中，为瘤病者也。"《灵枢·刺节真邪论》说："虚邪之入于身也深，寒与热相搏，久留而内着，……发于筋熘，……合而为肠熘，……为昔瘤，……为骨疽。"

在《内经》及以后历代中医文献中论述的许多疾病，诸如"石瘿""乳岩""失荣""噎膈""肠覃""癥瘕""积聚""痞气""崩漏"等病，《难经》中的"积聚"，《诸病源候论》中的"石痈""石疽""胫阴疽""石榴疽""肉瘤""肉疽""多骨疽"，《伤寒杂病论》中的"癥瘕"等，都是描述的位于肠、肝、皮肤、骨、子宫等各个部位的肿瘤。中医学历代文献中这些论述都是前人研究癌症的宝贵经验，对我们治疗癌症有指导意义。

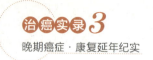

◇ 中医学对癌症的认识

中医的"癌"或"嵒"与岩通，是指体内发现肿块，表面高低不平，质地坚硬，宛如岩石而言。对于癌的发病认识，中医学认为主要是由于脏腑阴阳气血的失调，在正虚的基础上，外邪入侵或痰、湿、气、瘀等搏结日久，积滞而成。

《灵枢·百病始生篇》说："壮人无积，虚则有之。"这说明癌症的发生多在正虚的基础上产生的，特别是五脏的虚损尤为关键。由于七情、饮食失调等因素的长期作用于人体，使机体的阴阳失调，正气衰退，为癌症的生长创造了条件，而癌症的迅速发展，又进一步耗伤了正气，致令脏腑气血失调，同时更产生了一些病理性的因素，如痰结、湿聚、气阻、血瘀、郁滞等，与正虚并存，互为因果，形成恶性循环。

历代医家对肿瘤病因病机的认识及治疗有不同的侧重，或治病求本，或及于标，或及于脏腑，或及于气血，欲调其气、祛其邪、导其势而使其平。各家论述中有以为肝郁气滞者，如陈延之《小品方》"七气为病"之见；许浚《东医宝鉴》"六郁积聚"之论；虞抟《医学正传》"气郁湿滞，热郁成痰"之说；冯兆张《冯氏锦囊秘录》"理气为先"之治等。有以为气不能作块，而为食滞痰阻者，如朱丹溪《丹溪心法》"痰与食积死血"之说；戴思恭《证治要诀》"导痰汤"之治；陈士铎《石室秘录》"补气祛痰"之法等。亦有以为瘀阻内结者，其治如《金匮要略》大黄䗪虫丸、鳖甲煎丸，《黄帝素问宣明论方》鳖甲汤，《兰室秘藏》广茂溃坚汤等。有以为脾胃虚弱者，其治如《御药院方》蓬莪茂丹，《石室秘录》消补兼施汤，《鸡峰普济方》大白术丸等。有以为水湿不化者，其治如《仁斋直指附遗方论》温白丸，《丹台玉案》扶脾逐水汤，《宣明论方》三花神佑丸等。有以为阴虚内热者，其治如《石室秘录》软坚汤，《景岳全书》理阴煎等。

明代张介宾有"脾虚则中焦不足，肾虚则下焦不化"之论，并提出"大积大聚，如五积之久而成症病坚固不移者，若非攻击悍利之药，岂能推逐之乎！惟虚弱之人，必用攻补兼施之法也"之论；陈士铎《辨证录》"命门火衰不能化物"之说。叶天士《临证指南医案》倡久病虫类搜剔之治；李中梓《医宗必读》创"屡攻屡补，以平为期"之法等，不愧古今指南。王肯堂《证治准绳》论初、中、末三法，已说明对该病根据疾病的发展阶段而辨证施治的思想，如："初治积块未坚者，除之、散之、行之，虚者补之；……中治其块坚者削之，咸以软之，补泄叠相为用；……末治块消及半，住攻击之剂，因补益其气，兼导达经脉，使荣卫流通则块自消矣。"

孙思邈论述之"五瘿七瘤"，曰石瘿、泥瘿、劳瘿、忧瘿、气瘿，是为"五瘿"；肉瘤、骨瘤、脂瘤、石瘤、脓瘤、血瘤和息肉，是为"七瘤"。

古代医家认为癌症是一种全身性疾病的局部表现，与人体的五脏六腑、十二经络、奇经八脉都有着直接的关系。诚如《内经》所说："治病必求于本""邪之所凑，其气必虚"。癌症的病因可分为外因和内因。外因与感受外邪（包括各种外来毒素、致癌因素）有关；内因与七情内伤、饮食失调等有关。

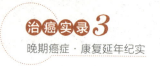

◇ **癌症的辨证**

中医对疾病的认识，绝不似西医那样，仅局限于局部的器官、组织、系统相应的病理改变，而在于生命的整体运动及其与全身阴阳气血的相互作用。癌瘤是身体严重的异常改变，虽然与外在环境因素、不良社会生活行为等有关，但主要为内在体质因素、生命运动方式变异等所致。对于病机的认识，不在定位、定性、定量，而在求因、求本，辨整体，审病势，看态势，概括病机以求其病变之源。注重脾肾为先天后天之本，脾阳不振，运化不及，导致突发异常改变；肾阳虚衰，控制失司，形成异常积聚癥瘕。审其趋势则有表里之分，求其势态则有病情发展的缓急之别，发展过程则有初、中、末之分。

◇ **致病因素**

癌症的发病原因虽然复杂，但可归纳为四类：①情志郁结；②脏腑失调；③饮食不节；④外感六淫。

七情（怒、喜、思、忧、悲、恐、惊）伤人之神气，心态的愤、恨、怨、恼、烦亦损伤阳气。癌症肿瘤发生于局部，但病因病机在整体，所以要采用整体观念和辨证施治，这是认识和诊治疾病的核心。无论什么癌，都要考虑全身气血的运行、五脏六腑的盛衰及相互的生克制化功能。

癌瘤的病因包括体质因素、血缘关系、遗传特点等常见的先天病因，时空、季节、致癌环境、六淫等特异的后天病因，情志心态、食饮劳逸等常见的后天病因。这些因素作用于人的生命过程，使各种运动方式的相互关系失和，并导致失通，于是这种异常的生命活动，便成为导致癌瘤的原因。

以外邪为例，六淫（风、寒、暑、湿、燥、火）伤人之形气。其中寒和湿为阴邪。阴邪伤阳气，如湿伤脾、寒伤肾；久湿困脾，则运化不及；久寒伤肾，则控制失司；另运化不及伤脾，惊恐久烦伤肾。其他诱因如大饮、过食、久劳、重力、淫乱、夜劳等均伤及脾肾。又五志过极皆能化火，情志过度，伐伤本脏，因而脾胃斡旋无力，气机不得条达，郁结积滞不通，日久则化火。其中喜、怒所致多为实火，而忧、思、恐、惊所致多为虚火。实属阳而虚属阴，虚火过盛则为阴火。

一般均认为癌症是在正虚的基础上发病的，表现局部为实，整体为虚。因此，应以正虚为本。在正虚脏腑阴阳气血失调下所产生的病变，如痰结、湿聚、气阻、血瘀、郁滞、毒聚等都属于标，基本属于正虚标实。从临床观察证明，未有仅具标实而正不虚的，即使是早期患者也有正虚的症状出现。

◇ 中医药治癌的特点

中医药在治疗癌症方面的特点有五：①阻止癌瘤增长；②减少其他治疗的毒副作用，提高抗癌效果；③防止癌瘤复发；④减缓癌症带来的痛苦；⑤中晚期癌症调理养生，力求长期

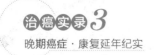

稳定。

《黄帝内经·素问》所述"坚者削之，客者除之，结者散之，留者攻之"，为早已确立的治疗大法。我们应当结合当今社会的特点，探索更为适宜的治疗方法。

中医药治疗恶性肿瘤的手段十分丰富，不仅有中药，还有针灸、气功、食疗等方法。根据临床辨证，以扶正为目标，或攻或补，或攻补兼施。祛痰、散结、化瘀、行血、通滞、攻毒，各种方法的记载具体而详尽，远比西医手术、化疗、放疗单一的攻击方法灵活优越得多。此外，用外治法治疗肿瘤也是中医药学的一大特色。外用抗癌药对于缓解疼痛、控制肿瘤发展也起到了一定的作用。

针灸作为肿瘤治疗的一种手段，可以调整阴阳失衡，增强抗病能力。气功则是强调内因的整体疗法，可以疏通经络，调理气血，平衡阴阳，达到改善症状、提高生存质量的作用。

生命修复可以治疗晚期肿瘤，更可以治疗早期肿瘤及癌前病变。尽管大量前来就诊的患者是晚期的，也有不少早期患者通过治疗取得了尽早切断其恶性发展，杜绝其进一步恶变及转移的良好效果。癌前病变常常表现为发病部位的细胞异常增生，虽无肿瘤却有明确病变等，例如食管上皮细胞重度增生与食管癌，萎缩性胃炎与胃癌，乙型肝炎、肝硬化与肝癌，子宫颈病变与子宫颈癌，黑斑与皮肤癌等，对于这些癌前病变积极治疗，阻断其恶性发展，可以将癌症消灭于萌芽之中，中医药在这方面有很好的临床效果。

◇ 中医临床上治疗癌症的常用方法

1. 祛邪扶正

祛邪和扶正是辨证治疗的两个方面。祛邪和扶正必须运用辨证的方法，辨别寒热虚实以进行合适的治疗。祛邪可以消癌，扶正也是为了消癌。祛邪和扶正相辅相成。

祛邪，一般根据致病之邪，如痰、湿、瘀、滞、积、聚、寒、火等邪，采用化痰、祛湿、化瘀、通滞、消积、软坚、温阳、清解、攻毒等治法，选用相关药物，以达消除毒邪之目的。

扶正，是运用补益药物增强机体抗病能力，根据气血、阴阳、脏腑的虚损，调整机体内部平衡，以达"正气存内，邪不可干"的效果，是治疗恶性肿瘤的重要环节。扶正与祛邪的主次是根据患者体质强弱、病程长短、肿瘤大小及早期、晚期等具体情况全面权衡而制定的。

攻补兼施，各脏腑均有虚实的不同，气血、阴阳亦有虚实的表现，治疗时需根据其具体情况辨证权衡。癌症患者免疫功能低下，一般认为攻补兼施属于非特异性免疫的范畴，二者合理配合可以减轻放疗和化疗的不良反应，保护骨髓造血功能，从而提高疗效，使得病情获得稳定。

在抗癌治疗过程中，有时会扶正与祛邪、攻与补同时应用。扶正与祛邪，同用或兼用，完全根据治疗患者的辨证需要而定。祛邪常根据不同的病邪，选用化痰、祛湿、导滞、散结、消积、解毒、攻毒等不同功效的中药。

常用培补虚损的中药有人参、党参、西洋参、太子参、当

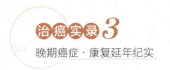

归、白术、山药、黄芪等。

2. 行气通滞

气与血是生命活动的重要物质基础，气为血之帅。《素问·调经论》说："人之所有者，血与气耳。"《景岳全书·血证》说："人有阴阳，即为血气。阳主气，故气全则神旺；阴主血，故血盛则形强。人生所赖，唯斯而已。"气有运行、生发、肃降、固摄、补益的作用，治疗方面则有行气通滞、行气活血、益气摄血等方法。在癌症的治疗中，行气通滞、疏肝理气是最为常用的方法。

患者常先有气滞不通，后有气血瘀滞，癌症疼痛也多与气血运行障碍及经络系统失调有关。

常用行气通滞的中药有：香附、郁金、青皮、陈皮、苏梗、砂仁、玫瑰花、檀香、川楝子、枳壳、枳实、三棱、莪术等。

3. 活血祛瘀

"气主呴之，血主濡之。"血是气化生的基础和营运载体，血为气之母。血液的主要功能是营养和滋润。血行脉中，运行全身，内至五脏六腑，外达皮肉筋脉，对各脏腑组织不断地供应营养和滋润以维持正常的生理功能。血液运行不畅会导致瘀血，如积血、留血、恶血、蓄血、干血、死血、败血等都是在肿瘤患者中经常见到的病症。活血祛瘀在祛邪治则中常用于有瘀血表现者，治疗需要权衡邪与正的关系来运用补正、祛瘀、攻瘀等法。

活血祛瘀作用机制与抑制肿瘤细胞生长和改善微循环有关。许多药物能减低血小板的凝聚性，使癌细胞不易在血液中停留、聚集和种植，从而减少转移。活血祛瘀可以增加血管的通透性，减少血液的黏滞性，并有利于药物、免疫淋巴细胞的穿透及血液循环的功能恢复正常，发挥抗癌作用，消除微循环障碍，增强免疫力。

常用的活血化瘀抗癌中药有红花、桃仁、赤芍、水蛭、丹参、川芎、蒲黄等。

4. 化痰祛湿

痰湿是人体津液代谢障碍出现的异常潴留现象，水分在体内的流动运行失控，以致津液停聚，或饮酒、奶酪、生冷等使脾胃运化失健而导致，痰湿是病理产物，也是癌瘤中常见的毒邪。

化痰祛湿用于治疗有痰湿、痰凝的患者，常见肿物质地较硬，按之不痛或有压痛，或推之可动，或盘牢不移。痰湿，多在脾虚的基础上发生。因此，在治疗上多与健脾药合并使用。

常用的化痰散结药中具有抗癌作用的有天南星、半夏、贝母、白芥子、皂角刺、猫爪草、黄药子、昆布、海藻等。

5. 清热解毒

清热解毒是祛邪治则中的一种治法。运用具有寒凉性质的药物解除热毒之邪，如治疗瘟疫、肿瘤热毒、火毒、疮疡、热深毒重等。对于有毒邪和热象的患者，可以针对不同部位和特点，选用相应的清热解毒中药。

很多清热解毒药具有抗癌作用，常用的有白花蛇舌草、半枝莲、鱼腥草、夏枯草、金银花、连翘、大青叶、板蓝根、七叶一枝花等。

6. 软坚散结

肿瘤多为有形之肿块，因此除上述各种治法之外，还应软坚散结以治其肿块。《内经》早就提出"坚者消之……结者散之"

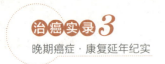

的治法，软坚散结使肿瘤先软化，再逐渐消散。

不通而肿瘤坚积。化结块，破坚积，散沉聚，宜峻药重剂。结而不坚者，以散结为主；结而坚者，以软坚为主。体虚者，不用推墙倒壁之力，而可用穿墙透壁之功。当正邪相持，邪强体弱时，宜用潜行钻透、开窍通关之品，搭配引泄毒邪、破结散积之剂。认明诸药相互作用的方向性，如根多升，果多降；花多升，叶多降；春采者多升，秋采者多降，借以引经通络，穿透攻坚，大气一转，其结乃散，此亦肿瘤的通治之法。组合运用化瘤、破结、散积之品，便可破坏肿瘤原有发生发展规律和肿瘤的生长方式，阻止其内外代谢交换，切断其营养供给途径。

常用的软坚散结药有牡蛎、鳖甲、山慈菇、海藻、昆布、僵蚕、穿山甲、夏枯草等。

以上常用治疗方法，不同于现代医学的单纯杀伤的治法。以各种方法杀死癌的思维是现代医学治疗癌症的主流，但这些方法不一定就是人类攻克癌症的唯一正确的方法。因为肿瘤细胞并非外来之物，而是自身体内生长出来的。由于肿瘤细胞的生命力远较正常细胞强盛，因此以杀伤细胞的方法来治疗肿瘤首先杀伤的是正常细胞、却不一定能杀死癌细胞，反倒会使它抗药、耐药、变异、加速生长、转移、恶化。

化疗药、放射治疗等已是非常强力的杀伤癌细胞的方法，这些尚且不能杀死癌细胞，因此我们就没有任何必要去重蹈覆辙，助纣为虐，对患者造成更大的伤害和打击。

生命修复采用中医中药治疗肿瘤，是集无毒、养生和健身为一体的治疗方法。

晚期肾癌双肺转移，周游列国 25 年

李女士 47 岁时患上肾癌，肿瘤很大，有 10cm。她在香港的医院作了一侧肾脏包括肿瘤的切除，但是几年以后发生了双肺的多发性转移。双肺大大小小的转移肿瘤有十多粒，当时医院和专家的评估都极不乐观，估计最多有几个月的生命。李女士到处奔走，去了香港、欧洲、美国等地就诊，希望能够找到有效的治疗方法，但是非常失望，所有地方的医生回答都一样，在这种情况下

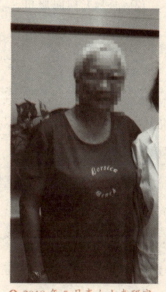

🎤 2018 年 5 月李女士来研究中心时留影

化疗、靶向治疗、放射治疗都不能够控制肿瘤的生长。无奈之下，李女士经朋友介绍前来用生命修复治疗。初来诊治时，她呼吸困难，气短不接续，胸痛咳痰咯血，生命垂危。

治疗原则

益肺填精，排毒消瘤。

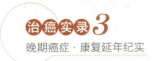

治疗方案

(1) 常用中药：人参、太子参、杏仁、北沙参、沙参、核桃肉、蛤蚧、天南星、石见穿、半夏等。

(2) 消瘤丸同时服用。

李女士一直坚持中医药生命修复治疗，取得了非常好的效果。如今她已经72岁了，自发展为双肺多发性转移的晚期癌症已有14年，从患癌算起已有25年。

晚期肾癌多处转移，尤其是双肺的大量转移，对目前的现代医学来讲，还没有确实有效的治疗方法。本案例患者肾癌肿瘤很大，手术切除以后，又发生了双肺的多发性转移，常规治疗的医师认为只能生存一年半载左右，但由于患者选择了正确的治疗方法，坚持不懈，长期抗癌，至今已正常生活了25个年头。特别是近年来，她到处旅游，去了中国的新疆、西藏、青海、北京、海南，还去了乌克兰、土耳其、巴西、阿根廷、智利、加拿大、摩洛哥及中东、南美洲等很多国家和地区，每次旅游返回，都会向我们介绍当地的风土人情，说她周游列国，一点也没有夸张。

附：患者相关检查报告

HISTOPATHOLOGY REPORT

Pathology No. _____

Previous Path. No. _____

Name ____ LEE ▨▨▨ ▨▨▨ ____ I.D. No. ____ ▨▨▨ ▨▨ ____ Sex/Age ___ F/47 ___ Date received ___ 8-3-93(20:55)

Hosp. or O.P.D. No _____ Ward/Bed No. ___ 735 (1) ___ Doctor _____

Specimen _____ Rt. kidney

Clinical summary/diagnosis
RUQ pain
Ultrasound & CT showed large tumour in Rt. kidney
Rt. radical nephrectomy done

GROSS DESCRIPTION

The specimen consists of a right nephrectomy weighing 438 gm. The kidney measures 13.5 cm. superior-inferiorly, 9 cm. medio-laterally and 7.5 cm. antero-posteriorly. It is surrounded by some fat. The attached ureter is 4 cm. in length. On sectioning, a large oval tumour is situated in the upper pole measuring 10 cm. at its greatest diameter. The cut surface of the tumour is yellowish with extensive haemorrhagic as well as microcystic degeneration. The tumour extends into the upper calyx dilating it. Some blood is seen in the lower calyx which is normal sized. No obvious tumour are seen in branches of the renal vein.
- (A) Transverse section of the ureter.
- (B) & (C) Represent one plane of sections taken from the hilum of the kidney.
- (B) Contain the tumour protrusion into the upper calyx.
- (C) Includes the renal vein.
- (D), (E), (F) & (G) Representative section of the tumour with (G) including the capsule.
- (H) Additional section of the hilum.
- (I) Represents the normal-looking kidney.

MICROSCOPIC DESCRIPTION

Section of the solid yellowish nodule in the centre of the lesion shows atypical cells with large hyperchromatic vesicular nuclei and prominent nucleoli. The cytoplasm is moderate and is either clear or amphophilic. These cells form small clusters and tubular structures surrounded by delicate fibrovascular stroma. This central solid nodule is surrounded by large cysts lined by cells with minimally enlarged and slightly hyperchromatic vesicular nuclei surrounded by abundant pinkish granular cytoplasm resembling oncocytes. The lumen of these cysts contains abundant proteinaceous material admixed with blood and has a microcystic appearance on gross-examination. The features are that of adenocarcinoma of the kidney (hypernephroma). The renal vessels at the hilum contain no tumour. The tumour is confined within the kidney. The capsule has not been penetrated. The rest of the renal calyx and pelvis shows mild chronic non-specific inflammation. Section of the ureter is unremarkable.

DIAGNOSIS

Nephrectomy (right) - Adenocarcinoma of the kidney.
- Tumour confined within the kidney with no invasion of renal vein.
- T_2, N_x, M_x.
- Assuming there is no lymph node and distant metastasis, this is stage II.

DATE ____ 10.3.93

○ 1993 年 3 月 8 日肾癌手术切除后，病理报告证实为肾腺癌

04-09-28 05:56 PM　　　　　　　HISTOPATHOLOGY　　　　　H 1

PATIENT'S NAME			DATE RECEIVED		PATHOLOGY NO.	COPY:
李■■ LEE ■■■■■■			16/09/2004		■■■■■■	DR. HOSP OTHERS
I. D .NO	SEX		AGE			
■■■■	P		58 Y			
HOSPITAL	HOSPITAL NO.	CLASS			PREVIOUS PATH. NO.	
■■■■	■■■	■■■			■■■	

UNDER CARE OF DR.

DOCTOR'S ADDRESS

CLINICAL PROCEDURE　　Core biopsies of 8 mm. nodule.

CLINICAL SUMMARY　　Carcinoma of kidney. Three small nodules 0.5 - 0.8 cm. in diameters.

FROZEN SECTION DIAGNOSIS (if any)　—

PATHOLOGICAL DIAGNOSIS

Lung (core biopsy) - Secondary adenocarcinoma.

REPORT

Supplementary Report

Immunohistochemical studies show the tumour cells are negative for TTF-1 (lung and thyroid), CK7 and CK20. The results would be more consistent with secondary adenocarcinoma from kidney, as diagnosed.

🎧 2004 年 9 月 16 日肺肿瘤病理检查证实为肾癌肺转移

Name:	LEE, ▓▓▓▓▓▓	ID No.:	▓▓▓
Sex/Age/DOB:	F/62▓▓▓▓	Room/Bed:	/
Ref.Dr.:	▓▓▓	Hospital No.:	▓▓▓
Exam ID.:	▓▓▓	Date of Exam:	23 Oct, 2007

LOW DOSE CT SCAN OF THORAX

<u>Clinical data:</u>
Ca kidney.

<u>Technique:</u>
One AP scout. 5 mm thick slices at 5 mm intervals through the thorax using low dose technique.

<u>Findings:</u>
Nodules of variable size are seen in the lungs. Their size and distribution are as follows:
1. R upper lobe, anterior subpleural region (0.28x0.22cm).
2. R middle lobe, medial aspect (0.56x0.22cm).
3. R middle lobe, anterior subpleural (0.39x0.28cm).
4. R lower lobe, medial aspect of posterior costophrenic sulcus (0.72x0.66cm).
5. R lower lobe, posterior (0.68x0.69cm).
6. L upper lobe, posterior (0.37x0.37cm).
7. L upper lobe, anterior (0.74x0.49cm).
8. L upper lobe, medial aspect (0.37x0.68cm).
9. L upper lobe, anterior subpleural (0.19x0.19cm).
10. L upper lobe, lingula (1.27x1.27cm).
11. L lower lobe, posterolateral subpleural (0.39x0.35cm).
12. L lower lobe, posterolateral subpleural (0.39x0.36cm).
13. L lower lobe, posterior subpleural (0.31x0.37cm).
14. L lower lobe, posterior subpleural (1.12x1.06cm).
For those that are tiny in size and subpleural in location, they are radiologically nonspecific.
For those that are bigger in size, given the clinical history of this patient, findings are suggestive of lung secondaries.

Two calcified granuloma are seen. The one seen in posterior subpleural region of L upper lobe measures 0.28cm in size. The one seen in apical segment of L lower lobe measures 0.17cm in size.

Mediastinum is clear. No lymphadenopathy is noted.

Hila appear unremarkable.

Imaged portion of liver and adrenals appear unremarkable.

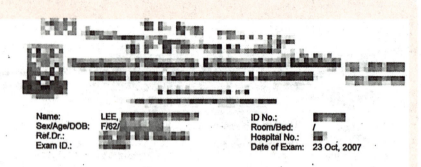

Name:	LEE,
Sex/Age/DOB:	F/62/
Ref.Dr.:	
Exam ID.:	

ID No.:	
Room/Bed:	/
Hospital No.:	
Date of Exam:	23 Oct, 2007

Impression:

1. Comparison is made with last low dose CT scan of thorax dated 27 Jul. 2007.

2. Multiple lung secondaries with extent as aforesaid. (N.B.: For those nodules that are tiny in size and subpleural in location, they are radiologically nonspecific.)

3. Two sizeable lung secondaries have mild interval increase in size:
a. L upper lobe, lingula
This now measures 1.27x1.27cm in size (last time, it measured 1.25x1.22cm in size).
b. L lower lobe, posterior subpleural
This now measures 1.12x1.06cm in size (last time, it measured 1.0x0.82cm in size).

4. The rest of the small lung secondaries show no significant interval change in size. No new lung secondary is noted.

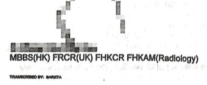

MBBS(HK) FRCR(UK) FHKCR FHKAM(Radiology)

TRANSCRIBED BY: @ARIZTA

♪ 2007 年 10 月 23 日 CT 检查报告证实有双肺和胸膜大量多发癌转移病灶

常见致癌因素

　　已知的导致癌症的因素大概有理化致癌因素、饮食因素、不良行为、环境因素、精神因素、遗传因素、水源污染、大气污染、生物毒素等。

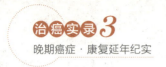

◇ **饮食因素**

饮食结构不正确包括进食不洁食物、变质食物、陈旧食物、不当加工的食物、腌制食物、不当发酵的食物，还有大量不当的肉类食品、刺激性食物、食物的防腐剂、不当的添加剂、合成色素等。当今的食物中采用的添加剂真是五花八门，种类繁多，如膨松剂、增香剂、嫩肉精、瘦肉精、增鲜剂、增稠剂、催熟剂、保鲜剂等，数不胜数，如果长期大量进食这样的食物会增加患癌的风险。

◇ **不良行为**

如长期抽烟酗酒，不良卫生习惯，不洁及不当的性生活等都会增加患癌的风险。

◇ **环境污染**

如汽车废气、工业污染、化工厂烟雾、放射性环境污染，如日本的核污染等。

◇ 理化致癌因素

接触有毒害的理化因素、滥用药物，特别是长期不合理地使用化学合成药物如性激素、各类激素、抗排异药物、解热止痛药物、抗癌药、止痛药、抗生素等。

◇ 精神因素

情绪长期压抑，紧张、悲伤、痛苦、愤怒、嫉恨等不良情绪也会增加患癌的概率。

◇ 遗传因素

家族中有患癌高发者也会增加患癌风险，但及早采取措施也是可以预防的。

对于其他未知的原因，我们通过多年来的临床经验分析和判断，也能深明其理，虽然许多研究和工作仍在进行，我们还是会在后文中提出一些预防癌症的忠告。

除以上列举的与癌症相关的因素之外，本书还选取了当今最普遍的又非常危险的，应予以充分重视而人们又视而不见的致癌毒素等问题，作为重点进行详细论述。

晚期脂肪肉瘤腹腔转移，愉快生活已 10 年

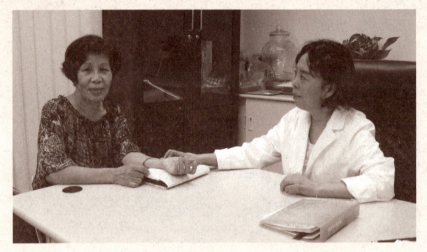

🔴 2018 年 7 月许女士在研究中心与医师合影

　　许女士于 2008 年 58 岁时，发现腹腔中有恶性程度很高的脂肪肉瘤并有双肺转移，她于 2009 年 2 月手术切除肿瘤，以后就来诊所长期服用中药。由于手术后医生及专家都认为，此种恶性肿瘤用化疗、放疗对肿瘤并无疗效，所以一直也没有做过什么化疗、放疗。许女士刚来就诊时并不能很好地配合。她当时认为自己只是患了良性的肿瘤，已经手术切除了，就没有必要治疗了，对于肺部转移病灶导致的咳嗽、多痰、胸闷等症状，她认为只是患了感冒气管炎。儿女们怕她担心而没有告知实情，使得她大意、轻视，更不愿意天天吃苦药。随着时间的推移，

她感到自己精神好转了，咳嗽改善了，又逐渐从家人口中得知这病的严重性，她才慢慢纠正自己的治病态度，配合治疗，成为一位颇有信心的抗癌斗士。

治疗原则

健脾益肾，祛邪攻毒。

治疗方案

(1) 常用中药：牡蛎、鳖甲、土鳖虫、桃仁、藤梨根、大黄、红参、山药、肉苁蓉、海藻、昆布等。

(2) 攻毒散同时服用。

时至今日，十年已过去，许女士一直生活愉快，也常来调理身体。

脂肪肉瘤属于软组织恶性肿瘤，由于本病血行转移者多，单纯手术切除不能预防复发、转移，化疗、放射治疗等效果很差。中医学认为本病属于"肉瘤""石疽""癥瘕""积聚"范畴。恶性肿瘤生长快，体积较大，浸润和破坏周围正常组织，并经常有广泛的血行扩散转移至肺、骨等。对许女士的治疗，以健脾益肾、软坚散结、祛邪攻毒并重。从整体出发和考虑，抓住积聚郁阻、毒邪为病的主要病机，从散结疏通、祛毒扶正立法，使患者恢复健康。

附：患者相关检查报告

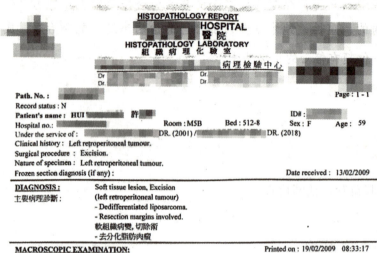

HISTOPATHOLOGY REPORT
醫院
HOSPITAL
HISTOPATHOLOGY LABORATORY
組織病理化驗室
病理檢驗中心

Dr.
Dr.
Dr.
Dr.

Page : 1 - 1

Path. No. :
Record status : N
Patient's name : HUI   許
Hospital no.:
Under the service of :   DR. (2001) /   DR. (2018)
Clinical history : Left retroperitoneal tumour.
Surgical procedure : Excision.
Nature of specimen : Left retroperitoneal tumour.
Frozen section diagnosis (if any) :

ID#:
Room : M5B   Bed : 512-8   Sex : F   Age : 59

Date received : 13/02/2009

DIAGNOSIS :
主要病理診斷：

Soft tissue lesion, Excision
(left retroperitoneal tumour)
- Dedifferentiated liposarcoma.
- Resection margins involved.
軟組織病變，切除術
- 去分化脂肪肉瘤

MACROSCOPIC EXAMINATION:

Printed on : 19/02/2009 08:33:17
(Patient discharged before issue of this report)

(MWP.)
Specimen consists of a large tumour with a smaller tumour attached together weighing 570 gm. The tumours have been cut opened. The large tumour measures 11.2 x 10 x 6.8 cm. It is covered by peritoneum on one surface. Cut surfaces of the tumour show myxoid whitish and yellowish tissue with focal haemorrhage and necrosis. The smaller tumour measures 2.6 x 2.3 x 2 cm. Cut surfaces of the tumour show myxoid whitish tissue. No calcification is detected in both tumours. The borders of both tumours are close to the excision margin. (A) Large tumour and its surface, 2 tissue blocks. (B) Large tumour and its deep margin, 2 tissue blocks. (C)&(D) Central part of large tumour, 4 tissue blocks. (E) Smaller tumour and deep margin, 2 tissue blocks. (F) Other parts of the smaller tumour, 2 tissue blocks. (G)to(M) 12 tissue blocks taken from various parts of the tissue. Figures 1 and 2 show cut surfaces of the large tumour. Figure 3 shows cut surface of the smaller tumour.

MICROSCOPIC EXAMINATION:

Section from the retroperitoneal tumour shows mainly proliferation of spindle cells in the stroma. The tumour cells show moderate to high grade cytological atypia. Some of the tumour cells show multinucleation. The cytoplasm of some of the tumour cells are eccentric with eosinophilic cytoplasm suggestive of rhabdoid differentiation. Mitosis is seen at 10/10 HPFs. Focal areas show myxoid change in the stroma with vague nodularity. In some of the myxoid area, there is proliferation of plexiform vascular structures. This area, however, is focal. In some areas, there is inclusion of adipocytes intermixed with the spindle cells. Some of the fat cells show cellular atypia with nuclear hyperchromasia and nuclear enlargement. Unequivocal lipoblast is not obvious. Some floret cells are noted. Lymphovascular permeation is not seen. Necrosis is present. Some foamy histiocytes are noted in the background. Some of the tumour cells show intranuclear inclusions. The spindle cells possess eosinophilic cytoplasm reminiscent of myoid differentiation. The tumour focally involves the resection margins. The overall features are those of a high grade sarcoma. In view of the presence of lipomatous component, the tumour is best classified as a dedifferentiated liposarcoma.

Date of report : 18/02/2009
jk

Approved signatory: ....

2009 年 2 月 13 日病理报告显示为去分化脂肪肉瘤

08 08 09 12:01   Dr ▓▓▓▓   23697009   p.1

Check and Medical Diagnostic Centre
醫學診斷中心

Name: HUI ▓▓ (許 ▓▓)	**General Line:**
HKID:	**Fax Line:**
Sex/Age: F / 59	**HKHCC ID:**
To: DR ▓	**Exam No.:**
	Date: 31/7/2009

EXAMINATION: CT Whole Abdomen (Upper + Lower) (Plain + Contrast)

Report:

CLINICAL INFORMATION:

retroperitoneal liposarcoma with excision/laparotomy in Feb., 2009, for progress

TECHNIQUES:

Pre and post contrast scan with arterial, venous and delayed phase
100mL Iopamiro 370 intravenous injection

FINDINGS:

Increase in density in the left perirenal space, along the inferior edge of the spleen and the left paracolic gutter. Features might represent post operative changes.

Both kidneys are of normal size and enhancement.
No evidence of hydroureters and hydronephrosis.
Spleen is of normal contour and size. No focal lesion identified.

Normal liver enhancement. Multiple hypodense lesions with no enhancement in all phase are present in both lobes of liver. Features are suggestive of multiple liver cysts. The largest one is present in segment VIII and measures 2.8cm x 2.8cm.
Normal enhancement of the portal vein and hepatic veins.
No evidence of intrahepatic duct dilatation. Gallbladder is of normal wall thickness. No gallstone identified. No evidence of pericholecystic fluid.

Pancreas shows no evidence of calcification. No focal lesion seen.
Normal caliber of pancreatic duct.
Bilateral adrenals are of normal contour and size.

Bowels are normal in caliber. No evidence of bowel obstruction.
No definite bowel mass identified.

COPY

No enlarged lymph nodes in the abdomen.
No ascites.

No lytic lesion identified in the bones.
Lung base covered in the examination show small lung nodules in both lung base (largest one measures 3.5mm in maximum diameter).

Printed: 31/7/2009 10:18:42   Page: 1

🎧 2009 年 7 月 31 日报告显示双肺有小的肿瘤结节

致癌毒素

毒素是什么呢？毒素是能够造成疾病的物质，也可泛指对人体有不良影响的物质。毒素可分为内源性毒素和外源性毒素。内源性毒素是指各种人体代谢产物，如自由基、尿酸、乳酸、酮酸等以及各种应该排出而仍滞留在体内的废物，如宿便、瘀血、痰浊、水液等。而外源性毒素则指大气污染、蔬菜中的农药残留、汽车尾气、工业废气、辐射、放射线、烟雾、化学药品、农产品中的防腐剂、化妆品中超标的重金属、过度煎炸、腌渍、过期的食物、垃圾食品等以及细菌、病毒、霉菌等病原微生物。

比如肠道的代谢产物如果停留太久，一些细菌能分解蛋白质，产生肽类、胺类、氨、硫化氢和吲哚等有毒物质。在正常情况下，它们被吸收进入血液，可在肝内转化、解毒，因而不损害健康。有毒物质蓄积日久，不能及时排出时，就可导致自身中毒。皮肤、脑细胞、肝等组织和器官都会受到毒素的危害。

　　西医认为的"毒"主要是指对人体有害的物质，包括来自外在环境的有毒物质和污染、细菌、病毒，及脂肪、糖、蛋白质等物质在新陈代谢过程中产生的废物。

　　而中医里"毒"的概念则更加广泛，不仅体内代谢出来的产物都叫毒，还包括机体所不能适应的"风、寒、暑、湿、燥、火"六大"病邪"。中医有解毒、排毒，攻毒等指的是通过全身调理来提高身体的适应能力，然后主动地将各种有害物质转化或分解掉，排毒方式包括排汗、排尿、排便、咳嗽、喷嚏等。

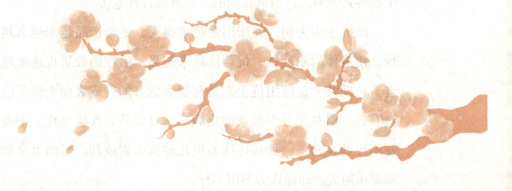

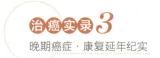

◇ 毒素的种类

有较大不良反应的药物以化学药品为代表，如类固醇药品、抗生素、镇静催眠药、止痛药等。

❋ 食物链的污染

农产品中的化肥、杀虫剂、残留农药等；渔牧肉品中的激素、抗生素、增长剂等；加工食品中的防腐剂、色素、添加剂等。

❋ 饮用水的污染

造纸厂、化工厂、开矿、养殖、施肥等对水源的污染。

❋ 大气的污染

汽车废气、火力发电厂、沙尘暴以及各种有害的物理、化学性物质污染大气，核辐射等污染。

❋ 内生毒素

人体新陈代谢后所产生的废物滞留，如粪便、二氧化碳、体内蓄积的重金属、自由基等。

❋ 生物毒素

包括致病微生物、病毒、细菌、霉菌、寄生虫等。大量的生物毒素能对人体造成长期的、严重的毒性危害。

以抗生素为例，临床用量越来越大，更新产品越来越多越快，使身体的耐药性、抗药性越来越强，治疗的效果也越来越差。长期及大量使用抗生素是有很大危害的，或表面上似乎已经有效，但往往会引起新的疾病。一旦停药，疾病恶化，则需要不停地换药，一种病往往要用几种抗生素或药。然而大家明知副作用大，却都认为不用不行。

◇ 宿便是内源性毒素的重要来源之一

人的身体也会产生毒素，比如便秘造成的宿便积蓄在肠道。按照症状不同，便秘可分为习惯性便秘和偶发性便秘两种类型。食物经消化吸收后在大肠形成粪便，这是身体向外排出毒素的主要途径之一。大便本来就是废物，粪便腐败后继续滞留在体内，会使大肠再度吸收毒素，并经肠道吸收进入血液循环，造成人体对已经排泄的毒素的再吸收。

如果毒存体内，则会影响脾胃的运行，造成大肠的传导失常，导致肠道不通而发生便秘。长期便秘导致粪便不能及时排出，便会产生大量毒素堆积，这些毒素被人体吸收，会继发肠胃不适、口臭等其他症状，导致人体器官功能减弱、抵抗力下降。

此外，宿便中的毒素被肠道反复吸收，通过血液循环到达人体各个器官和组织细胞，可导致面色晦暗无光、脸上出现色斑、皮肤粗糙、皮肤失去光泽、生暗疮等问题，还可引起便秘、腹胀、腹痛、痛经、月经不调、心情烦躁、口气难闻等症状。毒素作用于人体内酶系统，导致胶原蛋白酶和硬弹性蛋白酶的释放，这些酶作用于皮肤中的胶原蛋白和硬弹性蛋白并使这两种蛋白产生过度交联并降解，从而又使皮肤失去弹性，出现皱纹、松弛和过早衰老。

宿便中的毒素也会造成全身代谢、内分泌反常，五脏六腑功能障碍，继而引发各种不同疾病。

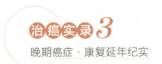
◇ 毒素积聚脏腑引起的疾病

1. 多种皮肤病

全身的皮肤是最大的排毒器官，皮肤上的汗腺和皮脂腺能够通过出汗等方式排出许多代谢废物。长期精神压力，内分泌紊乱，长期作息时间混乱，内、外源性毒素的危害，外界的不良刺激，内分泌障碍等，都会造成多种皮肤病，如皮炎、瘙痒、湿疹、痤疮、神经性皮炎、牛皮癣等。

(1) 黄褐斑：血行不畅，气滞血瘀，毒素堆积，会使内分泌发生变化，另外长期口服避孕药、肝脏疾病、肿瘤、慢性酒精中毒、日光照射等都能够造成黄褐斑的发生。

(2) 痤疮：痤疮是一种毛囊与皮脂腺的慢性炎症性皮肤病。各种毒素在细菌的作用下产生大量有毒物质，随着血液循环遍及全身，而当排出受阻时，又会通过皮肤向外渗溢，使皮肤变得粗糙感染而出现痤疮。精神紧张、内分泌失常、高脂肪或高糖饮食等因素也都会促使痤疮的发生。

(3) 湿疹：湿疹是因精神紧张或由环境中各种物理、化学物质刺激引起的皮肤长期瘙痒反应性疾病，另外，新陈代谢过程中产生过多的废物不能及时排出等也是湿疹的病因。

2. 消化系统疾病

(1) 肠道易激综合征：肠道对刺激有过度的反应出现，致使血流滞缓，排毒管道不通畅，多种毒素留存体内。发生腹痛、腹胀、腹泻、便秘等。

(2) 十二指肠溃疡：忧思郁怒、肝郁气滞的内生之毒，饮食不节、过饥过饱或过食辛辣等物，嗜烟酒带来的外来之毒等都可引起十二指肠溃疡。

(3) 口臭：口臭是指口内出气臭秽的一种症状，多由肺、脾、胃积热或食积不化所致，这些东西长期淤积在体内排不出去就变成了毒素。贪食辛辣食物或暴饮暴食，疲劳过度，感邪热，虚火郁结，或某些口腔疾病如口腔溃疡、龋齿以及消化系统疾病等都可以引致口臭。

3. 呼吸系统疾病

(1) 过敏症：如花粉热，过敏性鼻炎，常见的症状有鼻痒、喉咙痒、嘴巴痒、眼睛红肿、眼睑肿胀、流鼻涕、打喷嚏、呼吸道阻塞等。常见的过敏原有花粉、螨虫、灰尘、蟑螂、猫、狗、兔子等。

(2) 哮喘：许多环境因素与哮喘的发展和恶化相关。例如过敏原、空气污染和环境中的其他有害化学物质等。

4. 代谢系统疾病

(1) 结石症（胆、肾等结石）：环境因素、饮食不良、职业作业长期接触不良物质及体内毒素排出障碍等是引起结石症的主要原因。

(2) 尿酸、痛风、关节炎、风湿病：环境因素及体内毒素排泄障碍是导致痛风、关节炎等疾病的重要原因。

5. 心脑血管疾病

毒素堆积使体内毛细血管脆性增加，血管容易破裂，可诱发和导致心脑血管疾病的发生。宿便中的毒素进入血液还会导致中老年人出现高血压、心脏病、血栓性疾病、脑血管意外等

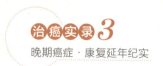
病。临床上因便秘而屏气使劲排便，从而增加腹压并造成心脑血管疾病发作，如诱发心绞痛、心肌梗死、脑出血、中风猝死等的现象有逐年增多的趋势。

6. 肿瘤

身体中肿瘤、癌瘤的存在是体内有毒素、废物堆积的明确表现，不论用什么方法治疗，排毒都是必需的。而排毒的具体方法则因患者的病情、身体状况及毒素堆积的部位等不同而不同。

7. 肥胖或瘦弱

太胖或太瘦都是新陈代谢异常所致。太胖者脂肪堆积，与代谢废物一起堵塞经络；太瘦者代谢废物造成消化吸收不良，无论怎样进食仍然消瘦。

清除体内垃圾可避免肥胖。体内"壅堵"会引起肥胖，而且这种肥胖是"向心性"的，即中间大两头小，状如枣核。这是因为废物久存体内，被人体重新吸收，造成了脂肪代谢障碍。另外，肠内垃圾不清除，在腐败细菌的作用下可产生大量气体，使腹部体积增大，腹围加大，久而久之，腹部肌肉松弛，腹部前凸形成向心性肥胖。这会影响女性的曲线美，也会使男士的"将军肚"日渐隆起。

8. 神经系统疾病及免疫力下降

毒素影响内分泌代谢功能。毒素也可以分布到神经突触和神经－肌肉接头处，直接损害神经元，造成中枢神经受损、身体各器官免疫力下降，出现经常性感冒、头晕、心悸、盗汗、失眠、健忘、注意力不集中、无缘故抑郁、四肢麻木等症状。

◇ 经络毒素蓄积的表现

1.肝经与胆经

《素问·六节脏象论》中说："肝者，罢极之本，魂之居也。"肝是最大的解毒排毒器官，其功能与调节精神情志、促进消化吸收以及维持气血津液的运行有关。胆经与肝经互为表里，互相影响。

肝胆经有毒素的表现如下。

(1) 指甲表面有凸起的棱线：是肝气郁结、体质变差、体力透支的征兆。一般有较长时间的精神紧张或睡眠不足、操劳过度或用脑过度。这是毒素在肝胆经蓄积的信号。

(2) 乳腺增生：乳腺位于肝经循行部位，肝郁气滞或痰气互结，瘀滞成块而发生肝经气滞痰结，影响了肝的疏泄功能，导致经前期胸胁胀满。如不及时治疗可能加重肝胆经的瘀阻，造成更多疾病。

(3) 悲观情绪：表现有自感精神压力、情绪低落、无精打采、悲观厌世、工作能力减退及厌食纳差等。肝脏是体内调控情绪的脏器，一旦肝内的毒素不能及时排出，阻塞气的运行，就会产生明显的不良情绪。

(4) 偏头痛：多发生在头部两侧肝胆经循行部位，还会伴有痛经（经期或经前腹痛）、胸胁胀满和急躁易怒等。

(5) 消化功能差：肝失疏泄会影响脾胃的升降和胆汁的疏布，从而出现肝胃不和、肝脾不调如食饮不振、腹胀、嗳气、消化不良等。

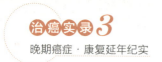

2. 心经与小肠经

心主血，开窍于舌，其荣在面色，与小肠经相表里。

心经与小肠经有毒素的表现如下。

(1) 舌头溃疡。心开窍于舌，舌和心脏的关系最为密切，所以舌头上出现溃疡，通常认为是心脏有火毒。

(2) 眼红目赤、口干舌燥、心烦易怒、面部疮痘等多为心火上炎之症。

(3) 心悸、失眠。心中悸动或惊恐不安，难于入睡，多梦，噩梦等，多为心经火毒之症。

(4) 胸闷或心痛。多为心血瘀阻影响心血心气运行的表现。

(5) 神志（精神）障碍。如神志悲伤、健忘狂躁等。

(6) 少腹胀痛、小便黄赤、小便不利等。

3. 脾经与胃经

脾胃是人体后天的生化之源，脾经转输水谷以散精气而营养全身，胃为水谷之海。

脾经与胃经有毒素的常见表现如下。

(1) 脾胃不调：多为饮食不节，中焦毒素积滞，呕吐呃逆、腹痛绵绵、不思饮食。

(2) 脾胃湿热：见脘腹胀满、身重体沉、大便溏泻、发热口渴等。

(3) 消化不良：见便秘腹胀、反胃呕吐、胃脘嘈杂等。

4. 肺经与大肠经

空气和食物都是生命的必需品。肺主气，司呼吸。大肠传导食物及糟粕，肺与大肠相表里。大肠经的毒素易于影响肺经，肺经的毒素也可以表现在大肠经。

肺经与大肠经有毒素常见表现如下。

(1) 皮肤晦暗：肺在体主全身的皮肤，皮肤的润泽要依靠肺的功能良好。当肺中毒素比较多时，毒素会随着肺的作用沉积到皮肤上，使肤色看起来晦暗无光。

(2) 便秘：肺脏和大肠相表里，当肺脏有毒素堆积时，可以通过经络表里关系影响到大肠内不正常淤积并出现便秘。

(3) 呼吸气粗：内、外邪毒袭肺，则呼吸气粗、咳嗽喘促、肌肤疼痛、寒热不调。

(4) 口干舌燥：肺经生寒热，则有口干舌燥、咽喉肿痛、咳吐痰液、胸痛引背等。

5. 肾经与膀胱经

肾与膀胱相表里，又与膀胱相通，膀胱的气化有赖于肾气的蒸腾，肾经的病变也会导致膀胱的气化失司。

肾经和膀胱经有毒素的表现如下。

(1) 月经问题：月经量少或经期短，颜色暗。月经的产生和疏导情况，可以体现肾功能是否旺盛，如果肾经中有很多毒素，经血就会异常。

(2) 水肿：肾主体内的水液运行，肾脏堆积毒素后，排出多余液体的能力降低，就会出现水肿。

(3) 容易疲倦：常见腰痛腿酸、形寒肢冷、头昏耳鸣、阳痿早泄、宫寒不孕、体倦、神疲思睡、四肢无力等症状。

(4) 排尿障碍：膀胱主行津液化水气，毒素堆积可出现尿急尿痛、尿浊、小便淋漓不尽、前列腺增生肥大等。

(5) 头痛、鼻塞、眼疾、颈背疼痛、腰酸腿软、转筋、痔疮、便秘等都属于肾与膀经循经所行毒素瘀阻可能造成的疾病。

从中医对疾病的认识来分析，毒素还包括了瘀血、痰浊、湿聚、寒气、食积、虚火、气滞等。这些毒素积聚在脏腑或者经络，会导致不同的疾病发生。

晚期皮肤癌腹腔转移，快乐生活 12 年

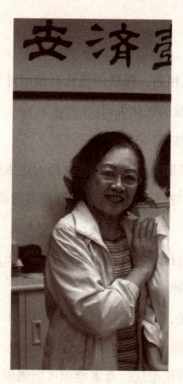

王太太是位喜爱运动的女士，特别是游泳，这是她多年的爱好。自退休后，她经常去海边游泳，然后躺在沙滩上晒太阳，当晒得出汗了，再跳进水里游一阵。

王太太于 2005 年经常腹痛，而且全身发痒，臀部又痛又痒，她当时并不是特别在意。但这些不适影响了她的游泳计划，她大半年来减少了许多运动。2007 年初她的病情加重，臀部

🔸 王太太于 2018 年 7 月来研究中心时留影

皮肤开始发硬并迅速溃烂。王太太这才急忙去看医生，非常震惊地得知自己患了皮肤癌，并且已经出现全身多发的淋巴转移，包括腹股沟及腹腔内、肠系膜等多处大量淋巴转移。医院确诊为皮肤癌第四期。

医院立即为她安排了手术，大面积切除臀部的皮肤。手术后愈合良好，接着又做了化疗，但化疗后，她感到疲乏无力，多处可以摸到的淋巴部位仍然肿大质硬，腹痛加重。医生告诉她，对于全身大量的淋巴转移已经没有治愈的办法，癌症还会复发，并且还会在全身多处出现。腹痛就是因为大量腹腔淋巴转移造成。生命最多能维持一年左右，让她想吃什么就吃什么。她不甘心就这样送命，于是前来进行生命修复治疗，当时她骨瘦如柴，精神疲惫不堪，失眠，腹痛严重，因为腹部肿块的压迫，下肢水肿严重。

 治疗原则

解毒化浊，软坚散结。

治疗方案

(1) 常用中药：白芥子、土茯苓、蜈蚣、全蝎、乳香、没药、猫爪草、夏枯草等。

(2) 消瘤丸同时服用。

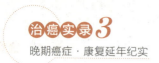

　　她每周都前来就诊，按时、认真地接受治疗，腹痛逐渐减缓、消失，面色转好，肿块消失，精神好转。如今，已经过去12年，她已有74岁，却一点也闲不住，还是积极参加各种社会活动并去游泳、唱歌。她完全康复了。

　　皮肤癌在中医学中有着不同的称谓，如"翻花疮""菜花"等。生命修复中医药治疗皮肤癌有一定的优势。首先我们认为局部性皮肤癌的手术治疗是不能解决根本性问题的。特别是已经发生了腹股沟、腹腔内、肠系膜等处大量的淋巴转移。局部的手术固然切除了癌瘤，但也只是暂时切除局部已破溃的以及更深层、更大一些面积的皮肤。切除对防止局部复发有利，但完全不能够治疗已经全身多处转移的病灶。如果没有进一步的生命修复中医药治疗，王太太的转移病灶会迅速发展，危及生命。所幸在手术之后，她选择了正确的治疗方法，控制住了大量腹腔中及肠系膜的肿瘤，使这些转移灶逐渐缩小直至消失。王太太现在大约两个月左右前来进行一次养生保健，正好上周她来，说中医药救了她的命，她将永远心存感激。

　　附：患者相关检查报告

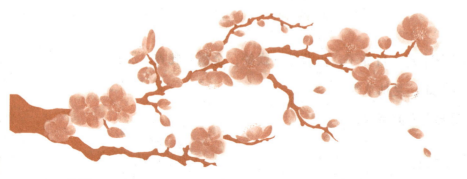

■■醫院 同位素及正電子掃描部

Department of Nuclear Medicine & Positron Emission Tomography

■■■■■■■■ HOSPITAL

Name:	Mak,■■■■■			Date:	25/4/2007
I.D. No.:	A11■■■■■	Sex:	Female	Fax:	
Hosp. No.:	■■■■■■	Age:	63 Y	Tel:	
Ward/Dept.:	■■■■■■				

POSITRON EMISSION TOMOGRAPHY
(^{18}F-FDG ONCOLOGY)

<u>History</u>:

A 63 year-old lady initially presented with 2 left groin masses. She was diagnosed sebaceous carcinoma of left buttock with excision done on 10/4/2007. One left groin node was excised and confirmed lymph node metastasis. Pre-operative CT scan showed a cluster of enlarged mesenteric lymph nodes up to 2.5 cm in lower abdomen and suspected of metastasis. PET scan for further investigation. DM on oral medication. No history of hepatitis or tuberculosis.

<u>Radiopharmaceutical</u>: 10.8 mCi F-18 Fluorodeoxyglucose (^{18}FDG) injected intravenously.

<u>Findings</u>:

Limited whole body CT transmission and PET emission imaging began at 46 minutes after radiopharmaceutical administration (blood glucose 6.8 mmol/l), spanning a region from vertex to toe. 60 mg Spasmonal was given p.o. 15 min before ^{18}FDG administration.

Liver tissue normal reference uptake has a SUVmax of 3.65 and delayed SUVmax of 2.66.

There are diffuse mild activities in the medial left groin and left buttock regions and likely represent post-operative inflammatory changes. A focally hypermetabolic left groin node is seen more laterally. The right groin appears normal with no abnormal lymphadenopathy. In addition, multiple enlarged hypermetabolic mesenteric nodes are identified in the lower abdomen with the largest one noted at L5 level. These are most consistent with multiple metastatic mesenteric lymphadenopathy. There is no abnormal uptake in the uterine and bilateral adnexal regions. The liver shows uniform uptake without any focal area of hypermetabolism. The adrenal glands and pancreas appear normal. The bowel shows some physiological activity. There is no hypermetabolic intramammary lesion in the breasts. Both lungs reveal no focal abnormal glycolysis. The mediastinum and bilateral hila show normal physiological activities. Bilateral supraclavicular and cervical lymph nodes are unremarkable. There is no abnormal uptake in the nasopharynx. Marrow activities within the axial skeleton are normal. No other suspicious hypermetabolic skin lesion is noted in the remaining regions of the body.

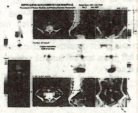

Functional parameters of these lesions are tabulated below:

Mak, Chui Ping	in cm			Standard	Delayed
Site	X	Y	Z	SUVmax	SUVmax
Liver (normal)				3.65	2.66
Largest mesenteric node at L5 level	1.9	2.4	2.0	3.81	6.57
Mesenteric node at S1 level	1.3	1.2	1.2	3.20	3.10
Lt groin node	1.0	1.2	1.0	2.52	2.92
Lt buttock activity	2.4	2.8	2.5	1.62	1.95

<u>Impression</u>:

1. Multiple metastatic lymphadenopathy are identified as left groin node and multiple mesenteric nodes in the lower abdomen.
2. Post-operative inflammatory changes in the left buttock and medial left groin regions.
3. No other metabolic evidence of solid organ involvement is noted.

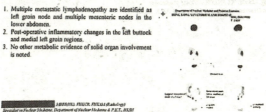

■■■■■■, FHKCR, FHKAM (Radiology)
Specialist in Nuclear Medicine, Department of Nuclear Medicine & P.E.T., HKSH

○ 2007 年 4 月 25 日同位素及正电子扫描报告证实：左腹股沟区有大量转移性淋巴结肿瘤，下腹部有大量转移性肠系膜淋巴结肿瘤

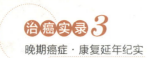

醫院 同位素及正電子掃描部

Department of Nuclear Medicine & Positron Emission Tomography

HOSPITAL

Name:	Mak,		Date:	3/8/2007
I.D. No.:	A1	Sex: Female	Ref. Dr.:	
Hosp. No.:		Age: 63 Y	Fax:	
Ward/Dept.:	Oncology		Tel:	

<u>Impression:</u>

1. Resolved mesenteric and left groin nodal metastases. As understood, metabolic quiescence is not equivalent to true tumoricidal effect. At least 2 serial PET studies demonstrating no abnormal metabolism may be considered more confirmative of metabolic remission.
2. Resolved previous post-operative inflammatory changes in the left groin and left buttock activity.
3. No new lesion is seen.

, MBBS(HK), FHKCR, FHKAM (Radiology)
Specialist in Nuclear Medicine, Department of Nuclear Medicine & P.E.T., HKSH

🎧 2007 年 8 月 3 日同位素及正电子扫描再次检查报告腹股沟及肠系膜转移性淋巴结肿瘤消失，连续 2 次 PET SCAN 检查未见异常

醫院 **Hospital** 醫院 **Hospital** 核子醫學部 **Department of Nuclear Medicine** 檢驗報告 **Examination Report**	Case No.: ▓▓▓▓▓ HKID: ▓▓▓▓▓ Name: MAK, (麥 Sex: **F** Age: **69y** DOB: **21/12/1943** Hosp / Spec / Ward: ▓▓▓▓▓	**R**

Imaging No.: ▓▓▓▓▓▓▓▓▓▓	Date : 11/01/2013 08:35

* DUPLICATE *

N
M

Examinations: WB Ca FDG, Delay Abdomen
PET-CT

Pharmaceuticals:
F18-fluorodeoxyglucose 360.29 MBq

Report:

CLINICAL INFORMATION
Sebaceous carcinoma of left buttock with multiple groin and mesenteric LN metastases in 4/2007. Given JF x 4 and follow-up PET showed CR. Last private PET in 4/2009 suggested re-emergence of disease over L. groin and 2 mesenteric nodes. On symptomatic care since then. For follow-up study.

PROCEDURE
Body weight = 51 Kg, Height = 1.51 m, Fasting blood glucose = 7.4 mmol/L
Radiopharmaceutical: 376 MBq [F-18]Fluorodeoxyglucose (FDG) IV
PET scanning: skull base to upper thigh at 60 min, abdomen and pelvis at 119 min
Plain CT for attenuation correction of PET data
Measurement of attenuation-corrected FDG maximum standardized uptake value (SUVmax)
Reference values: (i) Mediastinal blood-pool SUVmax 1.9; (ii) Liver SUVmax 3.0, delayed SUVmax 2.6

FINDINGS
Reference to report of last private PET on 17/4/2009.
Multiple enlarged mesenteric nodes are present, showing mild FDG hypermetabolism (largest 2.0x1.3cm, SUVmax 4.4, delayed SUVmax 4.9). These were present in last private PET study.
No hypermetabolic nodes in bilateral inguinal regions, or rest of abdomen and pelvis.
Subcutaneous scarring in left gluteal region with no FDG hypermetabolism.

Liver shows diffuse physiological activity with no distinct FDG-avid hepatic lesion.
No focal FDG-avid lesion in stomach, spleen, adrenals or pancreas.
Diffuse prominent activity along the large intestine, can be hypertonic activity, but small focal hypermetabolic lesion, if any, may be obscured.
Physiological activity in urinary system.
No hypermetabolic abnormality in uterus or bilateral adnexal regions. No ascites.

Pharyngeal and tonsillar activity are symmetrical and within physiological limits.
No focal FDG-avid lesion in the thyroid gland. No hypermetabolic cervical lymphadenopathy.

No focal FDG-avid lung nodule is present in both fields.
No pleural lesion or pleural effusion. No hypermetabolic mediastinal lymphadenopathy.

No focal FDG-avid skeletal lesion throughout the scanned range.

IMPRESSION
1. There are persistent mildly hypermetabolic mesenteric lymphadenopathies, which appear to have no gross interval change (with reference to last private PET on 17/4/2009). Please correlate clinically and follow-up reassessment as indicated.
2. No definite evidence of local cancer recurrence in left buttock, or recurrent nodal metastasis in left inguinal region.

	Reported by : Dr. ▓▓▓▓ on 22/01/2013 13:01

Report to   :
Requested by : ▓▓▓▓

Printed on   : 22/01/2013 13:01

Page 1 of 2

醫院	Case No.:		R
Hospital	HKID:		
醫院 Hospital	Name: MAK, (麥		
核子醫學部 Department of Nuclear Medicine	Sex: F Age: 69y DOB: 21/12/1943		
檢驗報告 Examination Report	Hosp / Spec / Ward:		

| Imaging No.: | Date : 11/01/2013 08:35 |

* DUPLICATE *

N
M

3. No other hypermetabolic metastatic lesion in this PET study.

Reported by : Dr. [ ] 22/01/2013 13:01

Report to :
Requested by :

Printed on : 22/01/2013 13:01

Page 2 of 2

⋂ 2013 年 1 月 11 日检查报告显示肿瘤无复发转移

滥用抗生素的危害

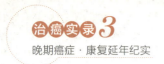

◇ 何谓抗生素

　　抗生素是抑制细菌生长或杀死细菌的化学物质。最先发现的抗生素都是由自然界的微生物所产生分泌出来的，例如100年前发现的抗生素——青霉素是由青霉菌所产生分泌的。这体现了自然界中物种之间互相制约、互生互灭的自然规律。后来研究人员则将这些原始物质的化学结构加以修饰改变，以化学合成的方式制造了许许多多不同结构的抗生素。目前可用来治疗人类细菌感染的抗生素有上百种之多。

　　不同的抗生素对细菌有不同的作用。有些抗生素可抑制细菌细胞壁的合成，有些可抑制其蛋白质的合成，有些则破坏其基因物质或阻断其新陈代谢的过程，因而造成细菌无法继续生长、繁殖，或直接使细菌死亡。人们找到各式各样的化学物质来抑制细菌的生长或杀死细菌这些物质同时也对人体内的生态环境产生了严重影响，导致内环境失衡，如破坏了肠道正常菌群。

　　在去看病就诊的时候，我们常可听到医师说："你需要吃抗生素或注射抗生素来治疗"，反之也有不少患者常会因感冒、咳嗽、喉咙痛或某某地方发炎而向医师要求开抗生素来吃，认为吃了这些抗生素，病症才会好。媒体也常有报道，如细菌对抗生素产生了抗药性，抗生素已经对细菌失效了。

　　侵入人体造成感染的微生物种类很多，有各式各样的病毒、细菌、霉菌、寄生虫等，因此当身体感染疾病，不一定全部都是抗生素能够治疗的，如果不管什么性质的感染全部都用抗生素，就会造成抗生素的滥用、乱用，这是导致身体耐药、抗药、疾病难愈以及抗生素不断更新换代等严重因素。我们应当意识到抗生素对于病毒、霉菌及寄生虫是没有作用的。此外，当身体某些地方有不适，或有炎症的时候，不一定就是微生物感染所造成的，例如关节炎就可能是因免疫功能异常损伤了关节组织而造成发炎，也可能因尿酸沉积过多而造成发炎，因此对于某些地方发炎也不一定就是抗生素的适用证。

抗生素不能称之为消炎药，因它本身并不具有直接消炎的效果，只有细菌感染所造成的发炎，使用抗生素杀死细菌后，才会使得感染部位的发炎减轻、消除。而非细菌感染所造成的发炎，使用抗生素是不可能达到消炎效果的。

◇ 细菌如何对抗生素产生抗药性

抗生素对细菌感染有效，有抑制细菌或杀死细菌的作用。细菌是单细胞生物，其分裂繁殖非常迅速，因此有相当的机会可以出现基因突变而衍生出不受抗生素作用的下一代。或抗生素原本定向作用于细菌的某一部位，但细菌的基因将该部位的结构改变了，使得抗生素无法作用于其上，因此细菌就不会被杀死；或者细菌的细胞壁结构发生了变化，造成抗生素无法穿透细胞壁，无法到达作用部位，细菌也因此不被抗生素杀死而存活下来。

这种不受抗生素作用、不被杀死的新生代细菌，在有抗生

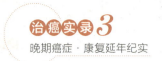

素的环境中也可以继续生长繁殖，我们称之为抗药性细菌，它们可存活下来并不断繁殖后代。长期以来，人们使用的抗生素愈来愈多，人体内一直在进行着细菌的对抗，这些筛选存留的抗药性细菌则可经我们的各种排泄物、分泌物释放到环境中或传播到其他人身上。因此，抗生素使用得愈多、愈普遍，抗药性细菌比例就愈来愈高。

◇ 细菌变成抗药性细菌后的影响

细菌对某些抗生素产生抗药性后，再遇到这些细菌感染时，这些抗生素治疗便无法将细菌杀死，细菌就在体内不断繁殖，从而造成越来越严重的感染。细菌最初对一、二种抗生素产生抗药性，尚可选择其他类的抗生素来治疗。但当细菌变成对大多数的抗生素或全部抗生素都具有抗药性时，就会产生严重的后果。

当今之所以会有这么高比例的抗药性细菌，就是因为抗生素一直滥用，相当于人们一直将非抗药性细菌逐步淘汰，而留存生命力顽强的抗药性细菌在环境中、人体内，一旦发生感染就非常难治疗。

随着抗生素在养殖业上的广泛使用，药物残留对人类生存的潜在隐患日益突出。除了因为"人用抗生素"过度使用以外，还有畜牧养殖业的滥用、乱用抗生素，例如养猪、养鸡、水产养殖等。饲养家禽家畜时，抗生素被大量的加入饲料中以促进生长或预防疾病发生，避免家禽家畜大量死亡而造成经济上的损失。部分抗生素还有对家禽家畜刺激生长的作用，因此这种做法会对在动物身上本来就存在的细菌产生筛选作用，衍生出对抗生素具抗药性的细菌，而这些抗药性细菌可能在我们进食时进入体内，造成抗药性细菌感染，经由此种途径传播到身体内，引起肠胃炎、菌血症、全身感染等。

另如，养殖场动物的粪便等并无适当的消毒处理，随着雨水、排水等途径流入江河湖溪。这些抗药性细菌将造成严重环境的污染，在环境中的抗药性细菌会很容易地进入人体，还可能造成动物身上的抗药性细菌基因传递给人身上的细菌，更加助长人体细菌的抗药性。

综上所述，细菌对抗生素的抗药性，基本上是人用及动物用抗生素滥用所造成的结果。明白这个道理后，我们就应不随便购买抗生素服用，不随意要求医生开抗生素来治疗各种各样的疾病。

◇ 使用抗生素的原则

对于抗生素的使用应该有以下几个基本原则。

• 抗生素对病毒及其他非细菌性的感染无效，一般感冒及流行性感冒是病毒性感染，而不是细菌性感染，不需要使用抗生素。

• 预防性地使用抗生素仅有在很少数的情形下有效而需要使用，大多数时候并不需要用抗生素来预防感染。

- 发热、发炎不一定都要用抗生素治疗。

- 合理选择使用抗生素，合理有控制地使用抗生素，有助于减少和控制抗药性细菌感染的问题。

- 不是什么病都需要先用抗生素，比如对肿瘤、癌症，抗生素是没有治疗作用的。

- 抗生素是有相当多副作用的药物，部分患者可能会出现过敏现象，少数患者也可能会出现一些其他的较严重的副作用，不是必需时，应避免使用抗生素。绝不可认为使用抗生素可以"有病治病、无病强身或预防感染"，尤其是若将细菌衍变成抗药性细菌后，后患无穷。

晚期肝癌复发转移，生意红火 12 年

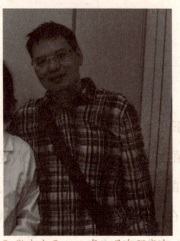

❶ 张先生于 2018 年 6 月在研究中心留影

张先生于 2004 年由血液查出乙型肝炎，尽管认真治疗，但 2005 年又发现有肝硬化，于 2006 年因消瘦明显、腹胀腹痛而去医院检查，肝癌指数 AFP 明显增高，又进一步做 CT 等检查，发现已患肝癌。张先生于 2007 年初做了手术，切除肿

瘤。此后做了一年的化疗，副作用很大，难以承受，但是他认为既然受了这么多罪，能够保以后平安也是可以忍受的。没想到化疗结束后，张先生于2008年去医院检查，肿瘤已经复发，肝脏又有新的肿瘤出现，并且得知，这种情况一般都是多发肿瘤，难以控制。

他当时每日感到疲惫不堪，腹部闷胀，食欲和消化均差。

通过朋友介绍，他前来接受生命修复的中药治疗，虽然路途较远，却风雨无阻。

 治疗原则

软坚散瘀，通滞攻毒。

治疗方案

(1) 常用中药：柴胡、白芍、鳖甲、丹参、石见穿、生大黄、玄明粉、土鳖虫、龙葵、山慈菇等。

(2) 消瘤丸同时服用。

经过一年多的治疗后，他的情况良好，连乙型肝炎指标也恢复正常，如今已12年过去，张先生一直健康快乐地经营着他的生意，他开了不止一家的餐馆，每日忙忙碌碌，高朋满座。

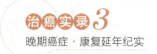

肝炎与肝癌有密切的关系，乙型肝炎与肝癌的关系更为密切，据有关报道，两者相关率高达80%，所以重视对乙型肝炎的预防和积极治疗是非常重要的。

治疗乙型肝炎是预防肝癌的重要手段。乙型肝炎若长期不能有效治疗，演变成肝硬化以后，随着病程进展，组织坏死修复的过程中容易发生基因突变，HBV增殖复制，可能导致部分患者最终发生肝癌。

生命修复和中医药在预防和治疗乙型肝炎，以及在治疗各阶段肝病、肝癌上疗效肯定，可有效控制癌组织生长和发展，对晚期患者和其他失去西医治疗时机的患者而言，中医药仍有很多机会和方法进行抗癌治疗。

附：患者相关检查报告

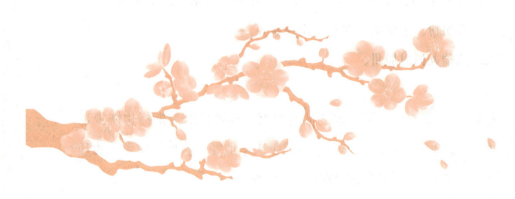

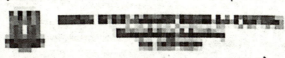

PATIENT'S NAME			DATE RECEIVED		PATHOLOGY NO.		COPY:
曾 ■■ CHANG ■■■■			20/01/2007		■■■■		DR. HOSP OTHERS
I.D. NO.	SEX		AGE				
■■■■■	M		39 Y				
HOSPITAL	HOSPITAL NO.		CLASS		PREVIOUS PATH. NO.		
■■■■	■■■■■■		■■■■		■■		

UNDER CARE OF DR.	■■ ■■■■■■ ■■■■■
DOCTOR'S ADDRESS	■■■■ ■■■■■■■■■ ■■■■ ■■■■■
CLINICAL PROCEDURE	Excision right lobe liver tumour.
CLINICAL SUMMARY	Segment 5 and segment 8 resection. Specimens segment 5, segment 8, gall bladder.
FROZEN SECTION DIAGNOSIS (if any)	---
PATHOLOGICAL DIAGNOSIS	(1) Right lobe liver (segmentectomy) - Moderately differentiated hepatocellular carcinoma, completely excised. (2) Gall bladder (cholecystectomy) - Benign.

REPORT

Macroscopic examination:

(1) "Segment 5 + 8 of liver" - Two pieces of liver tissue altogether 280 grams in weight, 12 x 9 x 5 cm., 7 x 5.5 x 4.7 cm. The larger piece, partly cut-open before receipt, showed a well-defined firm tan-coloured nodular tumour 3 x 1.8 x 1.8 cm. which was 1.1 cm. from the resection margin. The capsular surface of the liver was grossly intact. The smaller piece of liver tissue showed no definite macroscopic lesions on sectioning.

(2) "Gall bladder" - A green-brown smooth-surfaced gall bladder 7.5 cm. long, 3 cm. in diameter. On sectioning the mucosa was green-brown and intact and the wall measured 0.2 to 0.3 cm. thick. No stones were received.

Microscopic examination:

(1) Sections of the tumour show a moderately differentiated hepatocellular carcinoma with trabecular and focal pseudoglandular morphology. The tumour is multinodular, but no definite microsatellite foci are seen in adjacent hepatic parenchyma. Some dilated peritumoural lymphatics show tumour emboli without definite mural invasion. The capsular surface and resection margins are clear. Adjacent liver parenchyma shows an established cirrhosis, with minimal interface hepatitis, and extensive macrovesicular steatosis. The smaller piece of liver tissue shows no evidence of malignancy.

(2) Gall bladder shows no significant pathological abnormalities.

Date Reported: 22/01/2007

Signed: _____

Page 1 of 1

⋒ 2007 年 1 月 20 日肝癌病理报告，确诊为肝细胞癌

Name: CHANG,
Sex/Age/DOB: M/42/
Ref.Dr.:
Exam ID.:

ID No.:
Room/Bed: /
Hospital No.:
Date of Exam: 16 Dec, 2009

MRI SCAN OF ABDOMEN WITH AND WITHOUT CONTRAST

Clinical data: Ca liver resected.

Technique:
Pre-contrast:
Axial T1, T2, fat-sat T2, fat-sat T1
Coronal T2 weighted
Axial long fat-sat T2, in & out-of-phase

Post-contrast (Gadolinium):
Dynamic Axial fat saturation T1 weighted
Coronal fat saturation T1 weighted

Findings:
Comparison is made with previous MRI dated 26 May 2009.

Evidence of previous right hepatectomy is noted. Left lobe liver remnant is hypertrophied.

There is a small T1 slightly hyperintense and T2 isointense nodule in anterior aspect of left lateral segment. It shows signal loss in the opposed-phase image, suggestive of presence of intralesional fat. After contrast injection, no significant arterial enhancement is seen. It is hypoenhancing in the portovenous and delayed phase (series 16 image 40 and series 19 image 17). It is not seen in previous MRI.

No other focal mass lesion in the liver is demonstrated. Portal veins, hepatic veins and IVC are patent.

Bile ducts are not dilated. Spleen is not enlarged. No focal lesion in spleen is seen.

Both adrenal glands are normal. Left kidney is displaced inferiorly due to hypertrophied left lobe of liver. Both kidneys are otherwise normal.

No enlarged retroperitoneal lymphadenopathy is seen. No ascites is present.

Impression:
1. Status post right hepatectomy. Hypertrophied left lobe liver remnant.
2. Tiny fat containing nodule without significant arterial enhancement in anterior aspect of left lateral segment. It is not seen in previous MRI dated 26 May 2009. DDx include focal fat deposit, regenerative nodule or recurrent hepatocellular carcinoma. Suggest correlation with AFP and close follow-up MRI for progress.

Department of Diagnostic & Interventional Radiology
MBChB FRCR FHKCR FHKAM (Radiology)

2009 年 12 月 16 日检查报告，肝脏出现新生结节，以前的检查中没有，同时有 AFP 升高，肿瘤复发

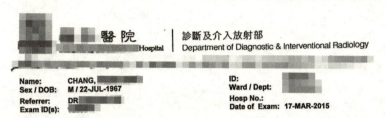

Name: CHANG,
Sex / DOB: M / 22-JUL-1967
Referrer: DR
Exam ID(s):

ID:
Ward / Dept:
Hosp No.:
Date of Exam: 17-MAR-2015

MRI SCAN OF ABDOMEN WITH AND WITHOUT CONTRAST

Clinical data:
Ca liver.

Technique:
Pre-contrast:
Axial T1, T2, T2 fat-sat, T1 fat-saturation
Coronal T2 weighted

Post-contrast (Gadolinium):
Axial T1 fat saturation
Coronal T1 fat saturation

Findings:
The right lobe of liver is absent consistent with previous right hepatectomy. Hypertrophy of liver remnant is noted. Reduced signal intensity of liver parenchyma is noted on opposed phase examination suggest fatty change. No abnormal mass is present. No abnormal arterial enhancing lesion to suggest hepatoma is present.
The biliary ducts are not dilated.
Portal vein is patent. No thrombosis is present.
The kidneys are normal in size and outline. No abnormal mass is present. No hydronephrosis is noted.
The pancreas is normal in appearance. No pancreatic lesion is present.
Pancreatic duct is not dilated.
Spleen is not enlarged.
Bowel structures have normal pattern. No abnormal bowel lesion is present. No obvious bowel mass is noted.
No significant adenopathy is present. No mesenteric adenopathy is noted.
No free peritoneal fluid is present.
Limited scan of both lung bases reveals no abnormal pulmonary masses.

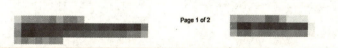 2015 年 3 月 17 日检查报告，肝脏没有肿瘤，全身无复发转移

畜牧业滥用药物的危害

◇ 抗生素残留对人的直接影响

通过食肉经常摄入的低剂量抗生素残留物会逐渐在体内蓄积而导致各种器官发生病变。抗生素的残留对人体的影响主要表现在变态反应、过敏反应、免疫抑制、致畸、致癌、致突变等方面。

如氯霉素（Chloramphenicol）可引起人类肝脏和骨髓造血功能的损害，导致再生障碍性贫血、血小板减少、粒细胞减少和肝损伤等；呋喃唑酮（Furazolidone）及其代谢物可使动物致癌。为此联合国粮农组织（FAO）、世界卫生组织（WHO）和美国食品药品管理局（FDA）均禁止在食用动物饲养过程中使用氯霉素和呋喃唑酮。

◇ 抗生素残留对人类的间接影响

抗生素的代谢途径多种多样，但大多数以肝脏代谢为主，经胆汁由粪便排出体外。一些性质稳定的抗生素排泄到环境中后会造成环境中的药物残留。这些残留的药物可通过畜禽产品直接蓄积于人体，或通过环境释放蓄积到其他植物中，并最终以各种途径汇集于人体，导致人体的慢性毒性作用和体内正常菌群的耐药性产生变化。

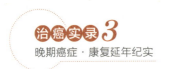
◇ 细菌耐药性对人类的危害

由于人们在食用动物的养殖中广泛应用抗生素，细菌耐药性的问题日趋严重和复杂。细菌耐药性不仅使抗生素的疗效降低，表现在药物剂量增大、疗程延长、复发率升高等，而且还会引起并发症，导致死亡率升高。全世界因食物污染而致病者已达数亿。

动物源性耐药细菌的耐药性向人类的转移，给人类的健康造成巨大影响，甚至威胁到人类的生命安全。尤其在动物中长期使用低于治疗剂量的抗生素可加速耐药细菌的出现。耐药细菌一旦在养殖动物中出现并在动物间传播，就可以通过直接或间接方式传递给食用动物的最终消费者——人类，对人类临床感染的治疗产生严重威胁。

大量抗生素被摄入动物体内后随血液循环分布于淋巴结、肾和肝等器官，使畜禽免疫力下降，病原菌乘虚而入则造成更严重的危害。长期、大量使用抗生素还会造成动物肠道内菌群失调，破坏微生态环境。

动物使用的抗生素主要以原形或代谢物的形式随粪、尿等排泄物排出，残留于环境中，对土壤、水源等生态环境带来不良影响，并通过食物链对生态环境产生毒害作用。

病案7

晚期甲状腺癌多发转移，操劳家务已9年

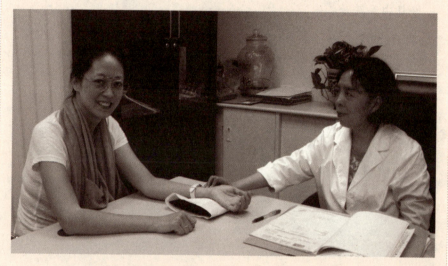

🔊 2018年7月孙女士来研究中心时与医生合影留念

　　孙女士于2009年33岁时发现患有甲状腺癌，并已出现双肺多发转移和全身多发性骨转移。她于2010年2月手术切除全部甲状腺及肿瘤周围组织。手术后病理报告证实，为乳头状甲状腺癌并向甲状腺周围组织扩散。切除的17个淋巴结中有14个已发生转移，左颈部组织切除的12个淋巴结中有8个发生转移，右颈部切除的组织中25个淋巴结中已有20个发生转移。手术后癌症的发展仍非常迅速，在2010年4月的CT显像检查中，发现右颈部和左锁骨都有多发的肿瘤结节，并有双肺转移，髂骨转移等多发转移灶，于是她又做了放射治疗。从发现晚期癌

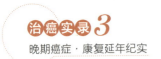
症后，在两年的时间内，她做完了所有要求做的治疗，如手术、放射治疗等，但是病情并不乐观，她的癌指数不断升高，转移灶不断增多、增大。无奈之下，孙女士前来求助于我们的生命修复中医药治疗。

她因骨转移而全身疼痛、无力并不停咳嗽，胸闷气短。

治疗原则

健中培元，祛邪攻癌。

治疗方案

(1) 常用中药：熟地黄、半夏、炙甘草、山药、杏仁、麦冬、百合、苏子、肉苁蓉、蛤蚧、牡蛎、重楼等。

(2) 消瘤丸同时服用。

自从用生命修复治疗不久，她的癌指数逐渐下降，转为正常状态，疼痛、无力、声音嘶哑等症状也在逐渐改善，从患晚期癌症全身多发转移至今已经九年过去了，她不想再去做那些有放射性损伤的检查了，因为她的生活很正常，每日忙于照料丈夫、女儿，帮女儿辅导功课，也常常带着全家一起去旅游。

附：患者相关检查报告

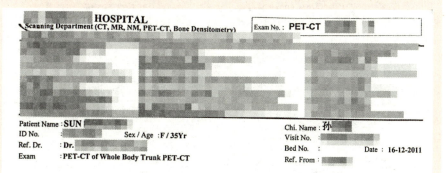

HOSPITAL
Scanning Department (CT, MR, NM, PET-CT, Bone Densitometry)

Exam No. : **PET-CT**

Patient Name : SUN		Chi. Name : 孙
ID No. :	Sex / Age : F / 35Yr	Visit No. :
Ref. Dr. : Dr.		Bed No. : Date : 16-12-2011
Exam : PET-CT of Whole Body Trunk PET-CT		Ref. From :

Clinical Information / History:

Ca thyroid with totally thyroidectomy done in February 2010. Multiple left neck lymph node metastases and bilateral lung and bone metastases at right ilium. 2 times radioactive iodine treatment. External RT to pelvis and thyroid bed given. Good general condition. Initially palpable left supraclavicular fossa lymph node was no long palpable. Chest X-ray clear. Serum thyroglobulin slowly rising.

Blood glucose level is 5.1 mmol/l.

Radiological Report:

RADIOPHARMACEUTICAL:

10.5 mCi F-18 deoxyglucose.

FINDINGS:

Whole body trunk PET-CT scan was performed from the base of skull to the upper thighs. Serial tomographic images of the whole body trunk were presented in transaxial, coronal and sagittal projections.

Evidence of total thyroidectomy is noted. No evidence of residual active tumour is noted in the thyroid bed. A prominent inactive lymph node is present at the left upper neck, measuring 7.5 x 7.5 x 12.1 cm. SUV max = 1.0, most likely reactive in nature. There is no hypermetabolic lymph node in bilateral neck and supraclavicular fossae. Focal uptake is noted at the left laryngeal area, near the posterior aspect of the left vestibular fold. SUV max = 4.6. This is a non-specific finding and may represent focal inflammatory, physiological uptake or less likely recurrent tumour. Endoscopic correlation is recommended.

NO. OF FILMS 10 14" x 17"			(DD-MM) (HH-MM)		
NO. OF COLOR PRINTS 18	NO. OF CDR 2	'WET FILMS: SENT		REPORT & FILMS SENT OUT :	
Remark :		RETURNED		16-12-2011	PM DHL

CHANYS

Report No. :

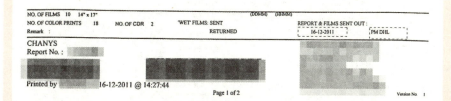

Printed by   16-12-2011 @ 14:27:44   Page 1 of 2   Version No. 1

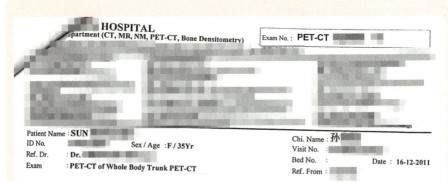

HOSPITAL
Department (CT, MR, NM, PET-CT, Bone Densitometry)

Exam No. : **PET-CT**

Patient Name : SUN

ID No.   Sex / Age : F / 35Yr   Chi. Name : 孙
Ref. Dr. : Dr.   Visit No. :
Exam : PET-CT of Whole Body Trunk PET-CT   Bed No. :   Date : 16-12-2011
                                                     Ref. From :

No active lesion is present in the mediastinum and hila. A 7.9 x 6.4 x 9.3 mm nodule is present in the left lung lower lobe apical segment. SUV max = 0.6, worrisome for early pulmonary metastasis. A tiny nodule is also present in the right lung lower lobe, that is too small for accurate characterization. This may represent a granuloma or early metastasis. There is no disease activity in bilateral breasts and axillae.

The liver shows uniform physiological activity. The spleen, adrenals, pancreas, GI tract and other abdominal and pelvic visceral organs are normal.

No active lesion is present in the axial skeleton. In particularly, no abnormal uptake is noted in the right iliac bone.

(SUV = Standardized Glucose Uptake Value.)

IMPRESSION :

No recurrent tumour is identified in the thyroid bed. No hypermetabolic lymph node is present in bilateral neck and supraclavicular fossae. Focal activity at the left laryngeal area may represent focal inflammation, physiological uptake or less likely recurrent disease. Endoscopic correlation is recommended.

Small nodule in the left lung lower lobe is worrisome for early pulmonary metastasis. The tiny nodule in the right lung lower lobe is too small for accurate characterization.

No disease activity is present in the abdomen and pelvis.

No active lesion is present in the axial skeleton.

Thank you for your referral.

(This examination does not include the brain.)

NO. OF FILMS 10 14" x 17"   (DDMM)   (HHMM)
NO. OF COLOR PRINTS 18   NO. OF CDR 2   'WET' FILMS: SENT   REPORT & FILMS SENT OUT :
Remark :   RETURNED   16-12-2011   PM DHL

CHANYS
Report No. :

Printed by   16-12-2011 @ 14:27:44   Page 2 of 2   Version No 1

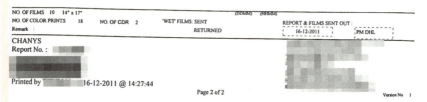
🔈 2011 年 12 月 16 日检查报告显示甲状腺癌伴大量颈部淋巴，双肺和多发骨转移

农药的危害

　　农药主要包括杀菌剂、杀虫剂和除草剂。农药对农业发展和粮食种植做出了贡献，然而随着农药长期大量的使用，农药残留及污染问题日益严重。据称，20 世纪 80 年代以来，大量施用农药带来的好处已被越来越多的危害所抵消。害虫杂草产生抗性，农药被迫越施越多，土壤质量下降影响农作物生长，各种生物和微生物均受到严重影响，与此同时也危害到了人类的健康。

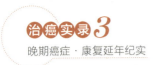
◇ 对人体的急性和慢性危害

急性中毒是严重的危害，据世界卫生组织和联合国环境署报告，全世界每年有 300 多万人农药中毒，20 多万人死亡。慢性危害表现在长期接触或食用含有农药的食品，可导致农药在体内不断蓄积，虽然不会立即出现严重的症状，但可以造成慢性损伤如破坏神经系统正常功能、破坏生育功能、影响免疫功能等。例如加拿大曾有食用杀虫剂污染的鱼和猎物致使儿童和婴儿出现免疫缺陷症的案例；德国在一项对儿童的检测中发现，新生儿体内农药残留超标；在对中国某城市哺乳期妇女的调查中研究人员发现乳汁中都含有微量杀虫剂。

◇ 严重污染土壤、空气和水源

据统计，农田中施用的农药量有 70% 左右扩散到土壤和大气中，导致土壤中农药残留量及衍生物含量增加，造成农田土壤污染。这不仅会破坏土壤中的生物多样性，还会通过饮用水或土壤 - 植物系统经食物链对多种生物和人体造成危害。

近年来，除草剂的增长率非常迅速。随着除草剂的大量施用，它对环境造成的影响也日益凸显。研究表明，在南非、瑞士、西班牙、法国、芬兰、德国、美国和中国等农药莠去津（Atrazine）使用历史较长的国家，地表水和地下水均受到了不同程度的污染。

　　杀虫剂最大的应用作物为果蔬，其他应用较多的有大豆、水稻、棉花等。多年大量使用农用杀虫剂，对环境造成了严重的污染。多种杀虫剂在土壤和空气中长期保持高浓度状态，土壤中残留的农药通常会随地表进入河流、湖泊，对地下水和地表水造成污染。杀菌剂主要用于水果、蔬菜、中草药等的病害防治。由于大部分杀菌剂在施用一段时间之后才可以看到明显的防治效果，因此它的使用剂量常被刻意提高数倍甚至数十倍，杀菌剂就成了重要污染源之一。欧盟早在 1996 年就指出，多种杀菌剂是农作物生产中主要的有害残留物。

◇ 对多种生物的危害作用

　　农药污染对土壤中微生物群落和多样性造成破坏，也对土壤中正常生存的动物如蚯蚓等造成不利影响。据不完全统计，在全世界已有 540 种昆虫和螨对 310 种化合物产生了抗药性。这对大自然生物多样性以及生物的自然生长造成了严重危害。进入水中的农药也会对水生生物造成毒害作用。

◇ 蔬菜水果等食品的严重污染

　　由于农药使用者缺乏农药知识和用药技术，他们长期大量不合理地使用农药会造成蔬菜、水果、畜禽养殖产品等农药残

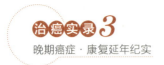
留量过高。农药和重金属是蔬菜、茶叶及粮食作物的主要污染物，据 2001 年统计，中国 23 个大中城市的大型蔬菜批发市场有 47.5% 的蔬菜农药残留超标。2012 年，叶雪珠等的调查指出，浙江省蔬菜生产中主要使用了 78 种农药，包括杀虫剂、杀菌剂、除草剂等。

◇ 致癌、致畸、致突变

有关流行病学调查显示，恶性肿瘤的发病率逐年飙升与蔬菜水果等食品中的农药残留有关，农药残留的毒性作用可导致胎儿畸形，这种力量远超过烟酒的危害。美国环保局证实，92 种以上的农药可以致癌，90% 杀虫剂有致癌作用。

2015 年国际癌症研究中心宣布：在动物实验中"有充足证据"证明剧毒农药草甘膦（Glyphosate）是致癌物（国际金融报，2015-05-04）。通过转基因种子捆绑草甘膦是致癌之源。国际癌症研究中心提示，伴随着转基因种子在全球种植面积增加，草甘膦除草剂使用量剧增。喷洒草甘膦后，只有针对草甘膦特性研发的转基因作物（玉米、大豆等）能存活，因此应用转基因种子就必须配套使用草甘膦除草剂。草甘膦致癌已引起有关部门的重视。

晚期恶性间皮瘤已9年，从生命垂危到成家立业

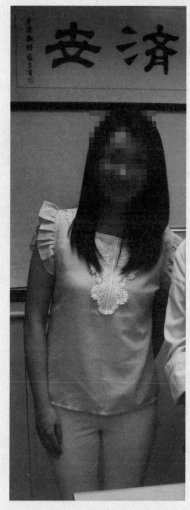

2018年7月贵小姐来研究中心时留念

贵小姐，2009年时只有21岁，一段时间以来经常有胸痛、腹痛，她以为是消化不良，没有当回事。以后胸痛、腹痛逐渐加重，腹部越来越大。她当时在澳洲留学，经在澳洲医院做病理学活检，确认为"恶性腹膜间皮瘤"，并已发生广泛的转移。当时澳洲医生认为病情危重，她即来香港，先来本诊所就诊2次，目的为先做好联系，介绍病情，以备手术之后有需要的话，可继续治疗。

她于2010年3月在澳洲医院手术，打开腹腔后，肿瘤严重扩散的程度令医生们感到震惊。因为腹腔中所有脏器全部都布满了大大小小、密密麻麻

的肿瘤，大如蚕豆，小如芝麻，已经占据了所有腹腔脏器。医生无法下手，不知所措，最后决定只能做一些选择性的切除，因为即使将腹腔器官全部切除，也难以全部清除肿瘤，况且也不可能这样做。手术切除了十二指肠、胆、脾和肝的部分及部分直肠和一侧卵巢。手术后 6 个月，查癌指数明显增高。再次做 PET 检查，显示腹腔中存大量肿瘤生长活跃，病情明显恶化。她即从澳洲返回香港，抓紧时间来做生命修复治疗。

贵小姐当时身体非常虚弱，腹痛严重，只能进少量流食。根据她的病情辨证施治，以扶助正气、攻邪抗癌为主要原则。她经常腹痛、腹泻，自手术后长期闭经，瘦弱不堪。

治疗原则

补正益气，攻毒抗癌。

治疗方案

(1) 常用中药：仙鹤草、鸡血藤、天花粉、薏苡仁、鳖甲、桃仁、重楼、田七、郁金等。

(2) 化癥丸同时服用。

　　她坚持来诊，风雨无阻，因为就诊看病的患者很多，家里为了让女儿休息好，父母经常大清早就来到了诊所，替女儿排队几个小时。她的父母也经常流着眼泪，询问还有没有希望。随着中医药生命修复治疗时间的延长，贵小姐越来越有精神了，腹痛慢慢消失，月经恢复正常，逐渐恢复健康。现在她工作、生活很正常，并于 2017 年 5 月结婚。9 年过去了，当时认为她活不过一二个月的澳洲医生，不得不对生命修复中医药刮目相看。

　　附：患者相关检查报告

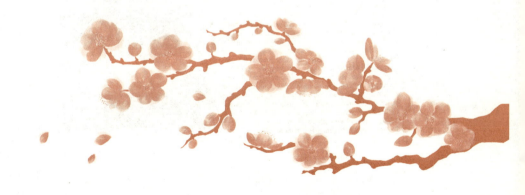

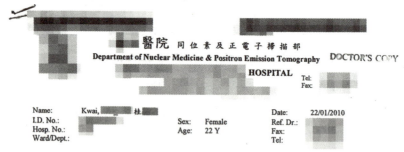

醫院 同位素及正電子掃描部
Department of Nuclear Medicine & Positron Emission Tomography DOCTOR'S COPY

HOSPITAL

Tel:
Fax:

Name:	Kwai, 桂		Date:	22/01/2010
I.D. No.:		Sex: Female	Ref. Dr.:	
Hosp. No.:		Age: 22 Y	Fax:	
Ward/Dept.:			Tel:	

POSITRON EMISSION TOMOGRAPHY
(^{18}F-FDG ONCOLOGY)

<u>History</u>:

A 22 year-old lady had a history of chest pain and palpitation in 09/2009. Blood test showed anemia, elevated CRP and ESR (>100), and elevated CA125 (2000+). MR of abdomen and pelvic was suspicious of hepatic parenchyma disease, with moderate ascites and small hypointense focus in the right ovary (suspicious for previous hemorrhage). Recently, she also noted midnight fever and skin rash. Gynecological sonogram was also suspicious of right ovarian thickening. She has no pelvic discomfort or distention otherwise. Non-diabetic, HBV negative.

<u>Radiopharmaceutical</u>: 10.1 mCi F-18 Fluorodeoxyglucose (^{18}FDG) injected intravenously.

<u>Findings</u>:

Limited whole body CT transmission and PET emission imaging began at 60 minutes after radiopharmaceutical administration (blood glucose 5.9 mmol/l), spanning a region from base of skull to upper thigh. 60 mg Spasmonal was given p.o. 15 min before ^{18}FDG administration.

Liver tissue normal reference uptake has a SUVmax of 2.17 and delayed SUVmax of 1.46.

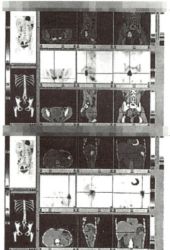

There is a moderate ascites within the pelvis. The uterus is deviated to the right. There is a slightly cystic focus to the right side of uterus suspicious to represent the right ovary. Behind this and on the right side of uterus, there is a curvilinear band of markedly increased glycolytic activity extending posteromedially and inferiorly towards the right side of Douglas pouch. This is suspicious for metastatic plaques along the right pelvis peritoneum medial to the right piriformis muscle. On the left side, there is also an intensely hypermetabolic lesion in the left side of pouch of Douglas, likely of the same pathology. Slightly below, there is a hypermetabolic left groin node, and slightly above, there is a hypermetabolic left external iliac node. There is little ascites in bilateral paracolic gutters, however, hypermetabolic lesions are detected adjacent to the caecum, lower descending colon, and intensely along the splenic flexure. These are most consistent with metastatic peritoneal plaques. In addition, discretely hypermetabolic lesion is seen anterior to the hepatic capsule of segment IV, consistent with right subphrenic peritoneal seeding. Minimal fluid is also noted within bilateral subphrenic spaces. No definite hypermetabolic pathology is seen within the liver (17.5 cm oblique height), bilateral adrenal glands, pancreas and spleen. Kidney configuration is normal. No definite

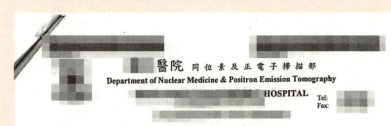

醫院 同位素及正電子掃描部

Department of Nuclear Medicine & Positron Emission Tomography

HOSPITAL

Tel:
Fax:

lymphadenopathy is seen within the retroperitoneum. Gastric activity is unremarkable.

In the thorax, there is normal parenchymal and pleural activity of bilateral lung segments with no lymphadenopathy in bilateral hila, mediastinum, supraclavicular fossae and jugular lymphatics. There is also normal activity of bilateral breasts and axillae. Marrow metabolism in the axial skeleton is within normal limits.

Functional parameters of these lesions are tabulated below:

Kwai, Wing Han	in mm		Standard	Delayed
Site	LD	PD	SUVmax	SUVmax
R POD mass	44.0	22.7	12.2	15.2
L POD mass	31.1	16.5	10.0	10.1
R subphrenic lesion	13.8	8.3	3.9	5.3
Peritoneal mass of splenic flexure	54.5	35.7	10.0	11.1
Lesion at or adjacent to caecum	18.0	12.4	7.3	10.1
L pelvic peritoneal lesion	27.6	10.0	4.6	5.6
A tiny focus adjacent to L iliac wing	14.0	11.3	3.0	2.7
L external iliac node	15.6	10.0	5.1	7.1
L groin node	12.5	11.3	5.8	8.5

Note: LD=longest diameter; PD=diameter perpendicular to LD

Impression:

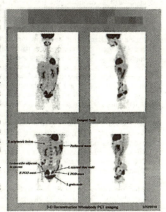

3-D Reconstruction Wholebody PET imaging 1/22/2010

1. Multifocal hypermetabolic peritoneal plaques are detected within the abdomen and pelvis. Together with ascites, these are most consistent with either a malignant infiltrative process or TB peritonitis. With elevated CA125, peritoneal carcinomatosis or lymphoma appears to be more likely than TB.
2. The largest peritoneal plaque is along right pelvic sidewall medial to right piriformis muscle and lateral to the uterus, extending into the right pouch of Douglas. The right ovary cannot be well delineated (except for vague hypodensity in the right adnexa). In view of these findings, right ovarian malignancy is suspected until proven otherwise.
3. Similarly, a smaller hypermetabolic mass is detected in the left pouch of Douglas and several hypermetabolic peritoneal lesions along bilateral paracolic gutters with a large peritoneal/omental plaque adjacent to the left splenic flexure of LUQ.
4. A hypermetabolic 1 nodule anterior to segment IV of liver represents a right subphrenic peritoneal deposit.
5. Hypermetabolic lymphadenopathy is identified in the left external iliac node and left groin.
6. No liver or extra-abdominal distant foci.

Thank you very much, Dr.

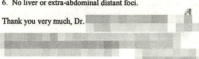

❶ 2010 年 1 月 22 日手术前检查报告显示大量肿瘤在膈下、脾曲、腹腔、盆腔、卵巢子宫后、髂部、腹股沟、盲肠等部位

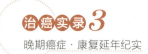

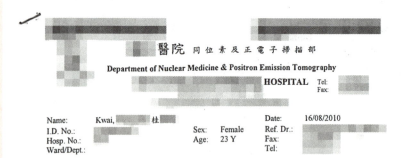

醫院 同位素及正電子掃描部

Department of Nuclear Medicine & Positron Emission Tomography

HOSPITAL Tel:
Fax:

Name:	Kwai, 桂			Date:	16/08/2010
I.D. No.:		Sex:	Female	Ref. Dr.:	
Hosp. No.:		Age:	23 Y	Fax:	
Ward/Dept.:				Tel:	

POSITRON EMISSION TOMOGRAPHY
(^{18}F-FDG ONCOLOGY)

<u>History</u>:

A 23 year-old lady had known malignant peritoneal mesothelioma with multiple ^{18}FDG-avid lesions on PET scan in 01/2010. She was treated with total peritonectomy, cholecystectomy, right salpingo-oophorectomy, splenectomy, diaphragmatic stripping followed by intraperitoneal chemotherapy with Alimta and DDP. Patient complained of vague right abdominal pain. Her CA 125 was elevated to 280. Non-smoker. Non-diabetic.

<u>Radiopharmaceutical</u>: 10.3 mCi F-18 Fluorodeoxyglucose (^{18}FDG) injected intravenously.

<u>Findings</u>:

Limited whole body CT transmission and PET emission imaging began at 71 minutes after radiopharmaceutical administration (blood glucose 4.7 mmol/l), spanning a region from base of skull to upper thigh. 60 mg Spasmonal was given p.o. 15 min before ^{18}FDG administration.

Liver tissue normal reference uptake has a SUVmax of 2.69 and delayed SUVmax of 2.28.

Patient is status post resection of peritoneal mesothelioma, splenectomy and right salpingo-oophorectomy. There is worsening over the active foci in right anterior subphrenic and left groin regions. New ^{18}FDG-avid foci are seen along the liver capsule, worst in right posterior subphrenic space near segment VII and beneath segment III. Patchy mild uptake is seen along the bowel (with more accentuated in transverse and sigmoid colon) and bilateral anterior pelvic cavity. The prior active foci involving the splenic flexure, adjacent to caecum, descending colon, bilateral POD and the left external iliac node are not seen. There is no definitive abnormal uptake inside the liver, bilateral adrenal glands, stomach and the uterus. No ascites.

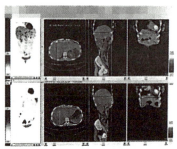

Mild swelling with obliteration of fossa of Rosenmüller is seen roof and posterior wall of right nasopharynx. There is diffuse increased ^{18}FDG uptake. The skull base above is unremarkable. No suspicious focal metabolism in clivus, petrous temporal bones and remaining sphenoid boned. There is no hypermetabolic lymphadenopathy in bilateral retropharyngeal spaces, jugular lymphatics, clavicular triangles, axillae, hila or mediastinum. Bilateral lung parenchyma reveals physiologic metabolism. There is no hypermetabolic intramammary lesion. No abnormal marrow uptake to suggest active osseous metastasis.

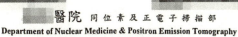

醫院 同位素及正電子掃描部
Department of Nuclear Medicine & Positron Emission Tomography

HOSPITAL Tel:
Fax:

Functional parameters of these lesions are tabulated below:

Kwai	Current Study Date (16/8/10)				Prior Study Date(22/1/10)				
	in mm				in mm				
Site	LD	PD	SUVmax	TLG	LD	PD	SUVmax	TLG	TLG% change
R subphrenic lesion	28.0	13.9	6.1	9.6	13.8	8.3	3.9	2.2	328.7%
L groin node	23.8	13.0	10.4	10.9	12.5	11.3	5.8	2.9	278.2%
Peritoneal mass of splenic flexure	Not active				54.5	35.7	10.0	103.6	-100.0%
Lesion at or adjacent to caecum	Not active				18.0	12.4	7.3	6.7	-100.0%
Bilateral POD mass	Not active				44.0	22.7	12.2	103.9	-100.0%
L external iliac node	Not active				15.6	10.0	5.1	4.2	-100.0%
New Lesion:									
Peritoneal focus beneath segment III	18.4	13.3	4.1	4.1					
Rt anterior pelvic cavity	13.4	8.2	1.5	0.5					
Sigmoid colon	32.6	23.9	3.1	15.1					
Transverse colon	22.3	10.8	2.8	5.8					
Rt nasopharynx	29.8	20.6	5.4	18.0					
Note: LD=longest diameter; PD=diameter perpendicular to LD; TLG=total lesion glycolysis (vol x SUVmean)									

Impression:

1. Post surgical resection of prior active peritoneal lesions in the splenic flexure, adjacent to caecum, descending colon, bilateral POD and the left external iliac node.
2. Worsening of active foci over right anterior subphrenic and left groin regions. Patchy activities around the capsular surface of liver, along the colon and bilateral anterior pelvic cavitiy are suggestive of active peritoneal disease. These may account for elevated CA 125 level.
3. Incidental findings of swollen right nasopharynx with increased ^{18}FDG activity. Correlation with nasopharyngoscopy and EBV DNA titre may be helpful to differentiate benign entity like focal nasopharyngitis from malignant pathology, or as clinically indicated.
4. No other ^{18}FDG-avid lesion in the remaining body survey.

Thank you very much, Dr.

⚫ 2010年8月16日手术后PET检查报告显示大量肿瘤恶化，活性增强。在膈下、腹腔、脾曲、盲肠、结肠、肝脏表面、盆腔、髂部、腹股沟等部位都有肿瘤病灶

寄生虫的危害

　　大多数人认为，只有贫穷落后的地区才有严重的寄生虫问题，但真相并非如此。当今，科学家鉴定出 300 种以上在美国大量繁殖的寄生虫，包括蛲虫、绦虫、钩虫、鞭虫、蛔虫等。美国有关部门曾报道，平均每一立方寸的牛肉里含有多达 1200 条寄生虫幼虫。估计 90% 以上的美国人遭受寄生虫问题却浑然不知，当症状出现时，寄生虫或许已在你身体内寄宿 10 年以上了。寄生虫是人体内的毒性媒介，是引发疾病和导致免疫系统功能低下的最基本原因。

◇ 食源性寄生虫的来源

寄生虫的来源有以下这些方面。

❋ **鱼源性**

以生食、食入未熟的咸、淡水鱼类感染的寄生虫。

❋ **肉源性**

以生食、食入未熟的动物肉类或动物内脏感染的寄生虫。

❋ **螺源性**

以生食、食入未熟的咸、淡水螺类感染的寄生虫。

❋ **甲壳类**

以生食、食入未熟的各种蟹或蝲蛄甲壳感染的寄生虫。

❋ **蛙、蛇类**

以生食、食入未熟的各种蛙、蛇类感染的寄生虫。

❋ **昆虫类**

以生食、食入未熟带虫的一些昆虫感染的寄生虫。

❋ **植物源性**

以生食、食入未熟的寄生虫污染的蔬菜、瓜果等感染的寄生虫。

❋ **宠物来源**

小动物的饲养，例如狗、猫等宠物身上的寄生虫传染给人等。

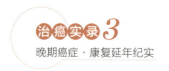
◇ 寄生虫对人的危害

寄生虫在人体的细胞、组织或腔道内寄生，会造成不同危害。

1. 夺取营养

寄生虫在体内生长、发育和繁殖所需的物质主要来源于宿主。寄生虫的数量越多，被夺取的营养也就越多。如蛔虫和绦虫在肠道内寄生会夺取大量的养料并影响肠道吸收功能，引起宿主营养不良；又如钩虫附于肠壁上吸取大量血液可引起贫血。

2. 机械性损伤

寄生虫对所寄生的部位及其附近组织和器官可产生损害或压迫作用。尤其有些寄生虫个体较大、数量较多时，这种危害是相当严重的。例如蛔虫多时可扭曲成团引起肠梗阻；棘球蚴（绦虫的幼虫）寄生在肝内起初没有明显症状，以后逐渐长大会压迫肝组织及腹腔内其他器官，发生明显的压迫症状。幼虫在宿主体内移行也可造成严重的损害，如蛔虫幼虫在肺内移行时穿破肺泡壁毛细血管可引起出血。

3. 毒性和抗原物质的作用

寄生虫的分泌物、排泄物和死亡虫体的分解物均有毒性作用，这是寄生虫所造成危害的重要方面。例如有些寄生虫侵入肠黏膜和肝时，分泌溶组织酶溶解组织、细胞，引起肠壁溃疡和肝脓肿；有的分泌排泄物可能影响造血功能而引起贫血。寄生虫的代谢产物和死亡虫体的分解物又都具有抗原性，可致敏，引起局部或全身变态反应，引起周围组织发生免疫病理变化，形成虫卵肉芽肿。有的抗原物质与相应抗体形成免疫复合物，引起过敏反应如过敏性休克，诱导宿主产生超敏反应，造成组织的损伤。还有许多寄生虫所产生的毒素危害尚未完全明了。

病案9

晚期唾液腺癌双肺转移骨转移，26 年抗癌史

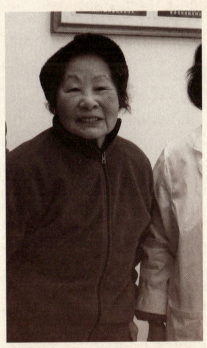

⬆ 陈女士于 2018 年 5 月来研究中心养生时留影

陈女士 77 岁，于 26 年前（即 1992 年）患头颈部腺样囊状癌，唾液腺恶性肿瘤，进行手术切除肿瘤，并切除部分下颌骨，还进行了下颌骨重建手术。至 2005 年肿瘤转移至右肺。2006 年她再次手术切除部分右肺，但又有新的肺部肿瘤，至 2015 年又发生了双肺的肿瘤和多发性骨转移。陈女

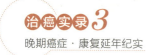
士年事已高，身体虚弱，难以再承受手术创伤。况且肿瘤已较为广泛地多发转移至双肺、肋骨、胸椎、腰椎等部位，也无法再进行手术切除了。无奈之下，她只有尝试用生命修复的中医药治疗。她当时气喘严重，呼吸困难，周身疼痛，咳嗽严重，头痛严重，有时神智不清，体弱病危。医院和家人都感觉到她的生命已经走到了尽头。陈女士开始时比较抗拒采用生命修复治疗，她认为反正已经无药可医，就没有必要再做任何治疗了，悲观厌世，疼痛不堪忍受。随着治疗的时间加长，她精神好转，疼痛从减轻到消失，咳嗽等症状也都明显改善到消失。

健脾补肾，祛邪消瘤。

治疗方案

(1) 常用中药：人参、鹿茸、补骨脂、桂枝、威灵仙、青龙衣、姜黄、桃仁、全蝎等。

(2) 消瘤丸同时服用。

　　陈女士最终改变态度，积极配合治疗，每次来就诊都笑口常开，还总是要求再增加一些针灸等辅助治疗，取得了很好的疗效。

　　明代医学家李中梓提出治病"初者病邪初起，正气尚强，邪气尚浅，则任受攻；中者受病渐久，邪气较深，正气较弱，任受且攻且补；末者病势经久，邪气侵凌，正气消散，则任受补"。患者虽是正气非常虚弱，却无法使用"只宜专培脾胃以固其本"的方法，全身大量转移的肿瘤特别是双肺的转移随时可能造成生命危险，所以祛邪、败毒、抗癌是必需的。选择解毒、补正与抗癌同时进行的方法，使得患者病情改善、痛苦日渐减少，越来越精神了。至今她患癌已有 26 年，今年 77 岁了，生活愉快，她自己说，一切都很好，也很快乐。

　　附：患者相关检查报告

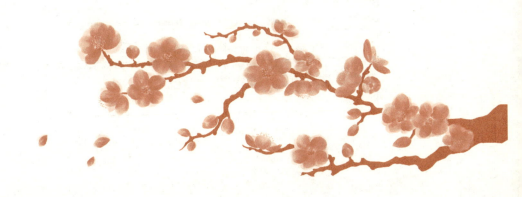

醫院 ███████
Hospital A████████
███ 醫院
P██████ M████████ Hospital
放射診斷科
Department of Radiology
電腦掃描檢驗報告 CT Examination Report

Case No.: ████ ████████
HKID: ████ ███ ███ ██████████
Name: CHAN, ████ ████ ███████
(陳███)
Sex: **F**   Age: **76y**   DOB: **1940**
Hosp / Spec / Ward: ████ / ████ / █████

Reg. Date: 06-Jun-2016 15:36

R

**C
T**

* DUPLICATE *

Procedure: CT neck, thorax, abdomen and pelvis

Clinical Information (from referring clinician):
History of adenocystic cancer of Head and Neck. Lung met resected 2006. Latest CXR shows 2 small lung nodules. For CT restaging

Diagnosis (from referring clinician):
Adenocystic CA of oral cavity with lung & neck LN relapses, resected & post-RT given. No evidence of disease.

Report:

CT neck, thorax, abdomen and pelvis:

Technique:
5/5mm NCCT and CECT

Findings:

Previous private CT dated 27/02/2016 is reviewed via ePR.

Neck:

Evidence of resection of right side of body of mandible with mandibular reconstruction. Evidence of previous right modified radical neck dissection.

Subcentimetre left sided cervical lymph nodes are seen, short axis measuring up to 0.8cm.

Cervical spine kyphosis, fulcrum at C5/6. Narrowing of C5/6 disc spaces with minimal retrolisthesis of C5 on C6. Posterior marginal osteophyte at C6. Short segmental ossification of posterior longitudinal ligament (OPLL) at C3, C4, C5 causing mild spinal stenosis.

Severe stenosis / occlusion of left vertebral artery at C6 level with distal reconstitution suggested.

Thorax, abdomen and pelvis:

Trachea and bilateral main bronchi are patent. No enlarged mediastinal or hilar lymph node. No pleural effusion.

Evidence of prior wedge resection in right middle (RML) and lower (RLL) lobes.

Reported by : DR. ████████████ ████████████ on 09-Jun-2016 21:36
Report to : ████████████
Requested by : ████ ████ ███ ███████
Generated on : 09-Jun-2016 21:36
Reprinted by ████████████ ████ on 04-Jul-2016 13:30

Page 1 of 3

醫院 ▓▓▓▓ **Hospital** ▓▓▓▓ ▓▓▓ ▓▓▓▓ **Hospital** 放射診斷科 **Department of Radiology** 電腦掃描檢驗報告CT Examination Report	Case No.: ▓▓▓ ▓▓▓▓▓▓ HKID: ▓▓▓ ▓▓ ▓▓▓▓▓▓▓▓▓ Name: CHAN, ▓▓▓▓ (陳▓▓) Sex: <u>F</u> Age: <u>76y</u> DOB: <u>1940</u> Hosp / Spec / Ward: ▓▓▓ / ▓▓▓ / ▓▓▓▓	**R**

▓▓▓▓▓▓ ▓▓ ▓▓▓▓▓▓ ▓▓ ▓▓▓▓▓▓▓▓▓▓▓▓	Reg. Date: 06-Jun-2016 15:36

C
T

* DUPLICATE *

Previously noted enhancing soft tissue nodules in superior segment of left lower lobe (LLL) and basal region of RLL, as well the subcentimetre nodules in apicoposterior segment of left upper lobe (LUL ; Se 9 Im 23) and lingula (Se 9 Im 36) show no significant interval change in size. Small LUL 8mm ground glass nodule (GGN) with a central 3mm soft tissue component (Se 9 Im 11) also shows no significant change in size. Another small 7mm GGN in central aspect of LUL (Se 9 Im 21) also shows no significant change.

Clusters of centrilobular nodules, some with tree-in-bud configuration, are seen in subpleural region of medial segment of RML. These can represent small airways disease or endobronchial infection.

Hepatic cysts and subcentimetre hypoattenuating foci in both hepatic lobes which are also probably cysts show no significant change. Prior cholecystectomy. Dilated central intrahepatic ducts and common bile duct likely related to post-cholecystectomy status. Pancreas and spleen are unremarkable.

Adrenals are not enlarged. Bilateral renal cysts. Tiny right renal stone. Collecting systems and ureters are not dilated. Urinary bladder is unremarkable. A 1.5cm rim-calcified lesion in right perivesical space can be phlebolith.

Prior hysterectomy and bilateral salpingo-oophorectomy. No abnormal pelvic soft tissue mass seen. No enlarged intra-abdominal or pelvic lymph node. No ascites.

Previously noted irregular cortical outline with mixed lytic and sclerotic changes in posterior left 7th rib associated with enhancing soft tissue along both inner and outer cortices shows no significant change. Patchy sclerosis in left scapula at region of glenoid, focal sclerosis in left posterior 8th rib (Se 5 Im 36), focal sclerosis in inferior aspect of right side of T3 body (Se 5 Im 13), and focal sclerosis in superior aspect of left side of L3 body (Se 5 Im 71) all with no associated cortical erosion or soft tissue components, show no significant interval change.

Impression:
1. Metastatic adenoid cystic carcinoma of head, status post-partial right mandibulectomy with mandibular reconstruction, right modified radical neck dissection, and wedge resection of RML and RLL, with:

- bilateral lung soft tissue nodules and subcentimetre left lung GGN which can be metastases, differential diagnosis includes lung primary with intrapulmonary metastases
- left 7th rib mixed sclerotic and lytic changes associated with enhancing soft tissue suggestive of metastasis
- patchy sclerosis in left scapula, focal sclerosis in left 8th rib, T3 and L3, these are non-specific

Reported by : DR. ▓▓▓▓▓ ▓▓▓ ▓▓ ▓▓▓▓▓ ── 09-Jun-2016 21:36	
Report to : ▓▓▓▓▓▓▓▓▓ **Requested by** : ▓▓▓ ▓▓▓ ▓▓▓▓▓▓▓	Generated on : 09-Jun-2016 21:36 Reprinted by ▓▓▓▓ ▓▓▓ ▓▓▓ ── 04-Jul-2016 13:30

Page 2 of 3

| 醫院
Hospital
醫院
Hospital
放射診斷科
Department of Radiology
電腦掃描檢驗報告CT Examination Report | Case No.:
HKID:
Name: CHAN,
（陳）
Sex: F   Age: 76y   DOB: 1940
Hosp / Spec / Ward: | R |

| | Reg. Date: 06-Jun-2016 15:36 |

* DUPLICATE *   C T

Overall findings show no significant change when compared with previous private CT in Feb 2016.

2. Clusters of centrilobular nodules, some with tree-in-bud configuration, in subpleural region of medial segment of RML. These can represent small airways disease or endobronchial infection.

Adverse reaction:
Nil reported.

| | Reported by : DR.   09-Jun-2016 21:36 |
| Report to   :
Requested by : | Generated on : 09-Jun-2016 21:36
Reprinted by   04-Jul-2016 13:30 |

Page 3 of 3

◐ 2016 年 6 月 6 日检查报告证实头颈部腺样囊状癌病史，于 2006 年曾切除肺部转移癌，又有新的肺部肿瘤。头部肿瘤术后下颌骨重建，双肺肿瘤（转移或原发）多发肋骨胸骨等转移

牙科填充剂有损健康

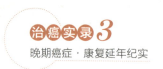

◇ 补牙材料的隐患和牙齿的健康

　　长期以来，牙医补牙时普遍使用银汞的补牙材料和含铅的材料，这些都属有毒重金属，对于人体是有危害的。以前的老观点认为单汞难以被人体吸收，但是新的研究发现，在咀嚼过程中微量的汞蒸汽会不断发散被吸收进入整个人体。如果是生育期的妇女应该特别小心，因为汞对胎儿发育危害很大。近年来，自闭症的孩子越来越多，研究认为与汞有重大关联。欧洲许多发达国家已经明令禁止使用银汞补牙材料，美国是建议谨慎使用含汞的补牙材料，而使用复合树脂等新的充填材料。现在有许多西方患者为了健康，甚至花钱把过去口腔里面的含汞补牙材料重新清除。但是，银汞的补牙材料在更多的国家目前却仍然大行其道，无人重视。

　　银汞主要是混合银、锡、铜及水银（汞）制成的。作为口腔修复材料，它有坚固耐磨、操作简便省时和价廉物美的优点。但由于银汞合金等材料中含有汞成分，人们越来越关注银汞合金的安全性问题。汞是目前已知的毒性最强的非放射性元素，汞可以在生物体内积累，很容易被皮肤、呼吸道和消化道吸收。吸入高浓度的汞会引发气管炎和肺炎并影响神经系统。在高浓度的汞环境中，肾功能会受到损害。牙科医生承认，当汞合金填充体被植入或取出时，会释放出汞蒸汽被人体吸收。虽然一些人认为，这种含量是微不足道的，但也不可完全忽视其对于健康的潜在危害。有些研究指出，汞与某些疾病有关，口腔中有汞合金填充体的患者患老年痴呆症的可能性更大。

美国食品和药物管理局（FDA）在 2009 年声明，银汞合金补牙材料中含有汞和其他金属，对于大多数成人和 6 岁以上的儿童是安全的。但在 2010 年，FDA 的科学家顾问团对银汞合金的补牙材料的安全性再次审查，敦促 FDA 继续审查和评估其安全性，表明这个问题还没有彻底解决。不管怎样，每个人要对自己的身体负责任，应该了解到这种潜在的风险。

◇ 现代化饮食导致牙齿疾病

美国牙科协会（National Dental Association）前主席 Dr. Weston Price（1870—1948）发现，牙科诊所里蛀牙与其他牙患者者日益增多，而生活在与现代文明隔绝的原始部落里的土著牙齿却特别好，牙病罕见。那些土著根本不知道刷牙为何物，也从未看过牙医。为了找到其中原因，他孜孜不倦，展开了艰难的探索之旅。他的足迹横跨世界，调查包括外赫布里底群岛、爱斯基摩、北美印第安区域的原住民、美拉尼西亚和波利尼西亚的南海岛民、非洲部落、澳洲原住民、新西兰毛利族以及南美洲的印第安等很多个部落。在对许多原始部落的调查中，Dr. Price 发现那些身体健壮的原始部落人具有漂亮、结实的牙齿，几乎看不见牙病，他们对疾病也有很强的抵抗力，而这一切源于他们传统的饮食。

与原始部落人的传统食物形成鲜明对比的是我们现代人食用的营养缺乏的食物：白糖、精米、白面、消毒的牛奶以及充

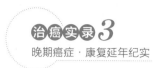
满各种添加剂的方便食品。

他在世界各地的调查清楚表明，现代人出现的龋齿、歪牙畸齿、牙弓发育不良是一种生理退化的标志，而其根源是现代食物缺乏营养。这表明随着人类社会的工业化，我们的食物营养结构与过去发生了巨大变化。

根据研究，Dr. Price 得出以下结论：健康的牙齿需要某些营养物质来构建。龋齿与牙病的主要原因是营养缺乏导致牙釉质形成不良、免疫力低下，以致逐渐被细菌入侵蛀蚀。原始部落的健康饮食提供了对龋齿的保护和抗病能力。人类从自然向现代文明过度，接受"现代商业食品"而造成了灾难性后果。现代人要想更好生存，必须把原始部落人的营养结构智能地融入现代生活方式。

但是，遗憾的是时间过去了七八十年，Dr. Price 的理论并没有得到足够重视，甚至可以说是处于尘封之中。原因非常简单，就是现代人已经无法回到过去那种简单而健康的饮食了。

晚期鼻咽癌加胃癌，战胜癌症17年

黎先生今年71岁，17年前患癌，当时他才54岁。

黎先生于2001年发现鼻咽癌，于2002年进行二个疗程的放疗加化疗，但是于2005年鼻咽癌复发并发生脊椎骨转移。他于2005—2006年做了手术，并又进行放疗以及化疗。但是这些治疗效果不好，肿瘤继续增大，癌指数增高，并出现头痛剧烈、呕吐，因而前来进行生命修复的中医药治疗。

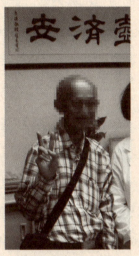

🎧 黎先生于2018年7月来研究中心养生时留念

 治疗原则

解毒化湿，散结消瘤。

治疗方案

(1) 常用中药：野菊花、鱼腥草、夏枯草、山慈菇、川贝母、浙贝母、僵蚕、牡蛎、蜂房、全蝎等。

(2) 化癥丸同时服用。

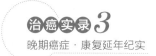

黎先生于 2007 年来进行生命修复的中医药治疗。此后他的病情逐渐稳定好转，由于曾经用大量的放射线治疗等原因，导致了听力受损，双耳聋。后又出现胃腹胀痛、恶心、呕吐等症状，他又进一步去检查，于 2012 年 8 月又查出胃癌。她又做了胃肿瘤的手术切除，手术之后，癌指数等仍然很高，医院要求再次化疗。根据以往的治疗经历，黎先生放弃了再做化疗、放疗等治疗，一直坚持生命修复的中医药治疗，至今他患鼻咽癌已 17 年，发展为多处转移的晚期癌症已 13 年，又患上两种癌已 6 年。但是现在黎先生已经康复，每日在室外运动、钓鱼，并帮助太太做家务。除了因为曾经的放射治疗造成的听力障碍之外，他没有其他不适，生活愉快。

化疗、放射治疗（电疗）的不良反应很多，这是大家都知道的事实。但是这些疗法的最大毒副作用就是有潜在的、使人体患上第二种癌症的风险。这一点其实是在不同的化疗等抗癌化学药物及放射治疗的说明书等之中已经有明确说明的。当前的癌症治疗，虽然使用了许多不同种类的化疗药、抗癌药物、标靶药物、免疫治疗等方法，但总的来说，患者的生存期并不是很长。也由于现在发现癌症以后在医院治疗的患者，多数都是中晚期，生存期不是非常长久，所以化疗、标靶、放疗等诱发第二种癌症的问题还没有引起足够的重视。

在我们的生命修复治疗中，患者的生存期得到明显延长。以前曾经做过化疗、放射治疗的患者患第二种癌症的可能性就成为值得注意的问题。目前，我们已经分析了这种情况，并且总结了继续用中医药治疗对化学药品和放射线所造成的癌症能够得到很好的治疗效果。也更进一步说明了，选择天然的、没有明显不良反应的方法治疗疾病和癌症有明显的优势。

附：患者相关检查报告

醫院 ████ **Hospital** ████ ██ 醫院 ████ **Hospital** 放射科 **Department of Radiology** 磁力共振掃描檢驗報告 **MRI Examination Report**	Case No.: ██ ████ **R** HKID: ████ ████ Name: LAI, ██ ██ (黎██) Sex: **M** Age: **61y** DOB: <u>25/11/1946</u> Hosp / Spec / Ward: ████

████ ████   Exam Date: 22/11/2008 11:50

* DUPLICATE *

Examinations: MR NP   **Contrast:**
Dortarem (20ml) 10.00 ml

REPORT:
Clinical History
NPC with RT in 2002
local relapse in 2006 with 2nd course RT and chemotherapy
clinically left V,VI,XII palsy
for reassessment

Clinical Diagnosis
NPC

Imaging Protocol:
Axial SE T1W, FS FSE T2W images
Coronal SE T1W images
Sagittal SE T1W images
Post-Gd coronal and axial FS SE T1W images

Imaging Findings:
(comparison was made with previous MR dated 29/1/06)

A thin 5mm layer of enhancing T1 hypointense, T2 hyperintense tissue is seen in Rt sided nasopharynx (SE2,3,6:16,17). This corresponds to the location of tumour in MR dated 29/1/06.
No extension across the midline is noted.
Mild increase in T2 signals and enhancement is seen in Rt pterygoid muscles and Rt infratemporal space (SE2,6:15), could be post irradiation change.
T2 hyperintense signals with slight enhancement (Se2,6:17) is seen in Lt parapharyngeal space.

The paranasal sinuses are filled with T1 isointense, T2 hyperintense signals with rim enhancement, likely represent sinusitic change. The opening of the Rt osteomeatal complex is markedly widened (SE4:17), ? post operative change. T2 hyperintense signals also noted in Rt mastoid sinus (Se2:19).

There is a ~1cm enhancing T1 hypointense, T2 hyperintense focus is noted at the base of odontoid (Se5:10)(Se2,3,6:8), similar to previous MR. However, the previously normal clivus is nearly completely replaced by T1 hypointense, T2 heterogenous hyperintense signals with patchy enhancement.
A 1.7x0.9x1cm (TDxAPxCC) enhancing T2 hyperintense lesion is seen just anterior to Lt sided clivus (Se6:16)(Se7:7), lying close to and nearly abutting the Lt ICA.

	Reported by : ████ ████ on 26/11/2008 12:38 ████ ████ 26/11/2008 13:35
Report to : ████ ████ **Requested by** : DR. ████ ████ ████	**Printed on** : 23/12/2008 11:08

Page 1 of 2

醫院管理局
Hospital Authority

■■醫院
■■■■ Hospital

放射科
Department of Radiology

磁力共振掃描檢驗報告MRI Examination Report

Case No.: ■■ ■■■■■■■   **R**

HKID: ■■■■■■■   ■■■■■■

Name: LAI, ■■■■■
(黎■■)

Sex: <u>M</u>   Age: <u>61y</u>   DOB: <u>25/11/1946</u>

Hosp / Spec / Ward: ■■■ ■■■ ■■■■

Exam Date: 22/11/2008 11:50

* DUPLICATE *

Enhancing T1 hypointense, T2 hyperintense signal is also noted in anterior C1 arch (Se2,3,6:12,13).

Loss of T1 bright signal is seen over the skull base of Rt middle cranial fossa with no abnormal enhancement associated, likely represent post irradiation changes.

The skull base is intact. No intracranial extension is observed.
No lymphadenopathy seen in the region included.

Impression:
1. Thin layer of enhancement in Rt sided nasopharynx, suggest correlate with endoscopy
2. Static enhancing lesion in base of odontoid, ? haemangioma or bone metastasis
3. New T2 hyperintense signals in the clivus and anterior C1 arch associated with patchy enhancement, ? post irradiation change or local invasion by tumour. Suggest follow up scan
4. New enhancing lesion anterior to Lt sided clivus, closely related to Lt ICA, ? local recurrence

Reported by : ■■■■■ ■■■■■ on 26/11/2008 12:38
■■ ■■■■■■ ■■ 26/11/2008 13:35

Report to : ■■■■■■■■■■   Printed on : 23/12/2008 11:08
Requested by : DR. ■■■■■■■■,
■■■■,

Page 2 of 2

◖ MR 检查报告显示 2002 年曾因鼻咽癌做过两个疗程的电疗和化疗，如今有复发及颅骨转移等

QUEEN MARY HOSPITAL

DEPT OF PATHOLOGY - Anatomical Pathology Division

A

HKID No:
Name: LAI,
Hosp No:
DOB: 25/11/1946
Sex/Age: M/65Y
Ref:

Hospital:
Lab No:
Queen Mary Hospital

Unit/Ward/Bed:
Request Loc:
Requesting Dr: DR.

Date Requested: 17/05/12
Date Arrived: 17/05/12

Final Report

CLINICAL HISTORY:
Gastric erosion (? malignancy) (535.40)
Epigastric pain, NPC, c/o epigastric pain + weight loss.

SPECIMEN(S):
Body.

GROSS EXAMINATION:
All embedded, 5 piece(s), 1 x 1 mm to 2 x 2 mm, 1 cassette(s).

MICROSCOPIC EXAMINATION:
Multiple sections show focally eroded body type gastric mucosa with moderately
active chronic inflammation. It is focally infiltrated by a poorly differentiated
adenocarcinoma comprising solid cords, poorly formed glands and occasional
signet-ring cells. The nonlesional tumor also shows intestinal metaplasia.
Helicobacter pylori are not found.

DIAGNOSIS:
STOMACH, body biopsy - ADENOCARCINOMA. ACTIVE CHRONIC GASTRITIS with INTESTINAL
METAPLASIA.

Reported by: DR P IP, MBChB FRCPath FHKAM(Pathology)
Authorized by: DR P IP, MBChB FRCPath FHKAM(Pathology)

Report Destination: QMH/--/%SRG - Department of Surgery

* Results subject to validation -- NOT FOR FILING   Page 1
Printed on : 01/06/2012 16:53:00

A

2012 年 5 月 17 日病理检查报告示：胃腺癌

醫院
Hospital
████████████醫院████ Hospital

核子醫學部
Department of Nuclear Medicine
檢驗報告**Examination Report**

Case No.: ████ ████████
HKID: ████████
Name: LAI, ████
（黎████）
Sex: **M**   Age: **69y**   DOB: **25-Nov-1946**
Hosp / Spec / Ward: ████████

R

N M

Reg. Date: 09-Nov-2016 07:54

Procedure: WB Ca FDG, Delayed Misc PET-CT, Delay Abdomen PET-CT

Pharmaceutical: F18-fluorodeoxyglucose 374.52 MBq

Clinical Information (from referring clinician):
Hx of NPC, choking, to rule out aspiration pneumonia, also noted elevated CEA and Ca 19.9, for PET-CT X R/O recurrence

Diagnosis (from referring clinician):
NPC, CA stomach

Report:

PROCEDURE
Body weight = 42kg, Height = 1.54m, Fasting blood glucose = 5.1mmol/L
Radiopharmaceutical: 375MBq [F-18]Fluorodeoxyglucose (FDG) IV
PET scanning: skull base to upper thigh at 60 min; abdomen at 130 min; neck at 140 min
Plain CT for attenuation correction of PET data
Measurement of attenuation-corrected FDG maximum standardized uptake value (SUVmax)
Reference values: (i) Mediastinal blood-pool SUVmax 1.8; (ii) Liver SUVmax 2.7

FINDINGS
Comparison with last PET study on 8/9/2015.
Previous total radical gastrectomy. No new focal FDG-avid lesion in the anastomotic site.
No new hypermetabolic abdominal or pelvic lymphadenopathy.
No new hypermetabolic peritoneal lesion or ascites.

Liver shows diffuse physiological activity with no new focal FDG-avid lesion.
Diffuse prominent activity in proximal ascending colon. FDG activity in rest of intestinal tract within physiological limits.
No new focal FDG-avid lesion in pancreas, other abdominal or pelvic viscera.

Previous bilateral apical fibrosis and mild atelectatic/fibrotic changes in left lung base similar. New mild atelectatic/fibrotic changes in right middle lobe with minimal activity. No other new focal FDG-avid lung lesion.
No new hypermetabolic mediastinal lymphadenopathy.
No new hypermetabolic pleural lesion or effusion.
Previous diffuse mild FDG activity along the oesophagus is also seen ?oesophagitis.

Previous right maxillary swing surgery. Previous patchy mild FDG activity in the sphenoid sinus and clivus with bony destruction is slightly less active with similar extent in this study (SUVmax 2.9; previously SUVmax 3.2).
Previous non-specific asymmetrical activity (SUVmax 3.2; previously SUVmax 3.0) in left side of lower nasopharynx similar. No new FDG-avid mass lesion in the nasopharynx or rest of pharynx.

Previous retention change in left maxillary sinus similar.

Reported by : DR. ████████ ██G on 22-Nov-2016 11:12
DR. ████████ ██ 22-Nov-2016 11:12
Generated on : 22-Nov-2016 11:12

Report to : ████████NPC
Requested by : DR. ████ ████ ████

Page 1 of 2

醫院 ▓▓▓	Case No.: ▓▓ ▓▓▓▓▓▓	R
Hospital ▓▓▓▓▓▓	HKID: ▓▓▓▓▓▓	
▓▓▓▓▓▓▓▓▓▓ 醫院 **Hospital**	Name: LAI, ▓▓ ▓▓▓	
	(黎▓▓)	
核子醫學部	Sex: M Age: 69y DOB: 25-Nov-1946	
Department of Nuclear Medicine	Hosp / Spec / Ward: ▓▓▓▓▓▓	
檢驗報告**Examination Report**		

▓▓▓▓▓ ▓▓ ▓▓▓▓▓▓▓▓▓ ▓▓▓▓▓▓▓▓▓▓▓ | Reg. Date: 09-Nov-2016 07:54

N M

No new focal FDG-avid thyroid lesion.
A mildly active right paratracheal node in lower neck is noted (~0.6cm, SUVmax 1.9). No new hypermetabolic cervical lymphadenopathy otherwise.

Focal mild activity in left posterior 9th rib, probably due to a fracture. No other new focal FDG-avid skeletal lesion throughout the scanned range.

IMPRESSION
1. Previous patchy mild activity in the sphenoid sinus and clivus with bony destruction is slightly less active with similar extent in this study.
2. A mildly active right lower cervical node in right paratracheal region is nonspecific ?reactive.
3. No other focal FDG-avid hypermetabolic lesion suggestive of a tumour mass, tumour recurrence or metastasis can be detected in this PET study.

Report to   : ▓▓▓▓▓▓▓
Requested by : DR. ▓▓▓▓▓▓ ▓▓▓

Reported by : DR. ▓▓▓▓ ▓▓▓ ▓▓▓▓▓ on 22-Nov-2016 11:12
                DR. ▓▓▓▓ ▓▓▓ ▓▓▓ 22-Nov-2016 11:12
Generated on : 22-Nov-2016 11:12

Page 2 of 2

⋂ 2016 年 11 月 9 日 PET–CT 复查鼻咽癌和胃癌，报告显示鼻咽癌及骨转移破坏均稳定无复发，胃癌无复发

提防辐射

◇ 我们身边的辐射

说起辐射，人们就会有些害怕，因为它看不见、摸不着，却会给人体造成伤害。其实辐射并不是一种稀罕物，我们的周围到处存在着辐射。在日常生活中，强烈阳光、过近距离看电视、戴夜光表、乘飞机、做 X 线检查等都会受到一定的辐照。只是生活中的辐照都是微量的，不会对人体造成伤害，所以人们也感觉不到它的存在。而大量的辐射对人体是非常有害的，因此我们应该通过采取一些相应的保护措施来防止和减少辐射对我们的伤害。

1.辐射对人体的效应是从细胞开始的

辐射会使细胞的衰亡加速，使新细胞的生成受到抑制，或造成细胞畸形，或造成人体内生化反应的改变。在辐射剂量较低时，人体本身对辐射损伤有一定的修复能力，可对上述反应进行修复，从而不表现出危害效应或症状。但如果剂量过高，超出了人体内各器官或组织具有的修复能力，就会引起局部或全身的病变。

2.日本核泄漏核辐射对人的危害

核泄漏的影响表现在核辐射，也叫作放射性物质。放射性物质可通过呼吸、皮肤伤口及消化道吸收进入体内，引起内辐射。γ 辐射可穿透一定距离被人体吸收，使人员受到外辐射伤害。

内外照射形成辐射病的症状有疲劳、头昏、失眠、皮肤发红、溃疡、出血、脱发、白血病、呕吐、腹泻等。有时还会增

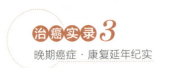

加癌细胞畸变，增加遗传性病变发生率，影响几代人的健康。一般来说，身体接受的辐射能量越多，其放射病症状越严重，致癌、致畸的风险越大。

核事故和原子弹爆炸的核辐射都会造成人员的立即死亡或重度损伤，还会引发癌症、不育、怪胎等。

◇　**放射性治疗的利弊**

医生和患者都有责任了解放射线的利弊。医疗放射的优势，在于能够检查出心脏、骨折、肿瘤等潜在问题，但也存在着严重的安全隐患。它损伤人的 DNA，可能在 10 ~ 20 年后诱发癌症。单独一项 CT（电脑断层摄影）扫描，其放射性就是普通 X 线射的 100 ~ 500 倍，据估计，美国有 1.5% 的癌症都因它而起。放射线治疗所用的放射剂量又远高于 CT 检查等，很多人也早就知道放疗、电疗会增加患者日后患上另一种癌症的风险，但医生们往往认为冒这个险是值得的。

◇　**注意电磁辐射污染**

要注意家居周围的电磁辐射是否超标。有不少家庭已经注意到自己所在的新建小区电磁辐射污染十分严重，不仅家里的电器受到过大干扰无法正常使用，而且许多人出现不同程度的不适症状。

这些电磁辐射对人体危害主要有以下几个方面。

(1) 它可能是造成儿童患白血病的原因之一。主要原因是距离高压电线太近。

(2) 电磁辐射污染会影响人体的循环系统、免疫、生殖和代谢功能，诱发癌症并会加速人体的癌细胞增殖。

(3) 影响生殖系统。

(4) 可导致儿童智力障碍。

(5) 影响到心血管系统。

(6) 对视觉系统有不良影响。过高的电磁辐射污染会引起视力下降、白内障等。

在日常生活中也要注意电磁辐射污染，不要把家用电器摆放得过于集中，以免使自己暴露在超剂量辐射的危险之中。特别是一些易产生电磁波的家用电器，如收音机、电视机、电脑、冰箱等更不宜集中摆放在卧室里。各种家用电器、办公设备、移动电话等都应尽量避免长时间操作，同时尽量避免多种办公和家用电器同时启用。手机接通瞬间释放的电磁辐射最大，在使用时应尽量使头部与手机天线的距离远一些，最好使用分离耳机和话筒接听电话。注意人体与办公和家用电器距离，对各种电器的使用应保持一定的安全距离，离电器越远，受电磁波侵害越小。

病案11

晚期胰腺癌腹腔转移，抗癌胜利已 8 年

胰腺癌是消化系统常见的高度恶性肿瘤，由于肿瘤生长速度和发展都极快，目前尚缺乏有效的治疗，一般认为其发病率与死亡率几乎相同，有"癌中之王"之称。西医通常会明确地告知家人此病的严重性，说明可做手术但预后不好，生存时间不长。

邓女士今年82岁，健康快乐，子孙满堂，享受着天伦之乐。但她是"癌中之王"胰腺癌的患者，患癌已八年了。

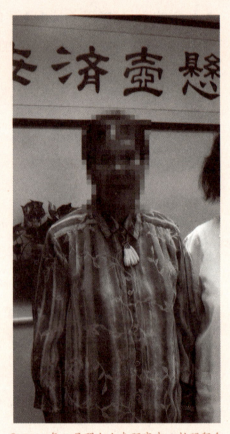

⚫ 2018 年 7 月邓女士来研究中心拍照留念

邓女士于 2010 年年初因腹痛不适、黄疸到医院检查，显示为胰腺癌，胰头已被广泛侵犯。她于 2010 年 10 月接受手术，因肿瘤大，要根据手术的报告考虑治疗方案。病理报告明确为

胰腺癌，手术前检查还有心脏增大。当时情况危重，腹痛严重，恶心呕吐，不能进食，全身黄疸。

正如所料，术后病理检查报告显示为晚期胰腺癌，病情严重，很不乐观。胰头部全部侵犯，肿瘤已包裹、侵入门静脉，并已侵入十二指肠固有肌层和周围神经。更没想到的是，一般手术切除肿瘤时会尽量多切除一些周围的正常组织，以免肿瘤切不干净，但是邓女士的检查报告显示，切除的癌瘤范围不足够，肿瘤距离切缘仅有 0.01cm，就是说切下的癌瘤周围并无正常组织，而有些部位更是没有切除干净。这种情况下，肿瘤复发和转移会在手术后很快发生，病情危重。医院和医生都认为她仅有最多几个月的生命，没有必要再受罪做化疗和放射治疗了。

家人经过一番了解和查询后，得知胰腺癌的化疗和放射治疗也并无明确效果，于是下决心不做化疗和放射治疗了。邓女士在家人陪同下前来中心进行生命修复抗癌治疗。她于手术后1个月余即来治疗，当时腹痛严重，不能进食，消瘦，呕吐。

 治疗原则

温运中焦，化毒消瘤。

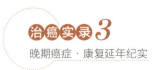
治疗方案

(1) 常用中药：牡丹皮、鳖甲、桃仁、干姜、砂仁、白蔻仁、
鸡内金、山慈菇、炮山甲、青龙衣、白芍等。
(2) 消瘤丸、化癥丸同时服用。

经治疗后，邓女士的病情明显好转，腹痛也逐渐缓解，进食增多，体重渐增，慢慢恢复了正常生活。多年来，每年去复查都未见有复发和转移，邓女士自诊断患有胰腺癌至今已有八年了，她生活愉快，与儿孙一起住，尽享天伦之乐。时至今日，邓女士战胜了"癌中之王"胰腺癌，但她从来没有做过任何化疗、靶向治疗或是放射治疗，她只是正确地选择了生命修复的中医药治疗。

附：患者相关检查报告

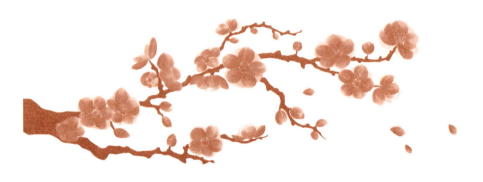

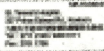

HISTOPATHOLOGY REPORT
HOSPITAL
醫 院
HISTOPATHOLOGY LABORATORY
組 織 病 理 化 驗 室

病理檢驗中心

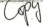

Path. No. :   Page : 1 - 1

Record status : B

Patient's name : TANG   鄧   ID# :

Hospital no. :   Room :   Bed :   Sex : F   Age : 73Yr10M

Under the service of :   DR. (1823)

Clinical history : Carcinoma of head of pancreas with portal vein encasement. Presented with obstructive jaundice.

Surgical procedure : Whipple's operation and resection of portal vein.

Nature of specimen : 1) Common bile duct resection margin. 2) Pancreatic resection margin; 3) Pancreatic duct. 4)
Whipple's specimen with portal vein marked by stitch.

Frozen section diagnosis (if any) : Please see below. (Kch.)   Date received : 10/11/2010

DIAGNOSIS :   1to4)   Head of pancreas, Whipple's operation
主要病理診斷：   (head of pancreas tumour)
(with excision of common bile duct resection margin, pancreatic resection margin and
pancreatic duct resection margin)
- Well to moderately differentiated adenocarcinoma.
- Tumour involvement of the muscularis propria of the duodenum.
- Tumour encasement and involvement of the portal vein.
- Focal perineural infiltration present.
- No lymph node metastasis (0/4).
- Close to adventitial resection margin (<0.01 cm).
- Focal perineural infiltration present in the pancreatic resection margin.
- No tumour involvement or dysplasia present in the pancreatic duct margin.
- Gastric remnant and duodenal resection margins clear.
胰頭, 輝普耳氏手術
- 高至中分化腺癌
- 參看下文

 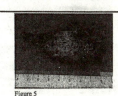

Figure 4   Figure 5

MACROSCOPIC EXAMINATION: Printed on : 12/11/2010   11:38:55

(KCH, jw)

Frozen section diagnosis - 1) Clear margin. 2) Mild dysplasia present. 3) Negative.

(KCH, yi)

1) CBD resection margin. Submitted is a ring of tubular structure measuring 1.5 cm across to the thickness of 0.4 cm.
All embedded for frozen section. Figure (1) shows the submitted specimen.

(KCH, jw)

2) Pancreatic resection margin. A piece of pancreatic tissue measuring 2.3 x 1.5 x 0.3 cm is submitted. All embedded
for frozen section. Figure (2) shows the submitted specimen.

to be continued ......

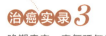

Path. No. :　■■■■　　　　　　　　　　　　　　　　　　Page : 1 - 2

Patient's name :　TANG ■■■ ■■■　邓■■　　　　　ID# : ■■■■■■

(KCH, il)

3) Pancreatic duct. Submitted is a piece of congested tissue measuring 0.5 cm long with a width of 0.2 cm. All embedded. Figure (3) shows the submitted specimen.

(KCH, yi)

4) Whipple's specimen. A Whipple's specimen is submitted. It consists of a gastric remnant measuring 6.2 x 3.3 x 1.2 cm and a segment of duodenum measuring 16.5 cm long with a diameter of 2.7 cm. The pancreas attached measures 4 x 5.5 x 2.3 cm. The two ends of the portal vein have been indicated by two surgical stitches. The mucosal surface of the gastric remnant and the duodenum are unremarkable. Cut surface of the pancreas show a yellowish ill-defined tumour mass of 3.9 x 3.5 x 3.2 cm located in the pancreas which is close to the resection margin measuring less than 0.1 cm away from it. The tumour shows no infiltration into the duodenal wall. Focal haemorrhage are noted in the tumour. The portal vein appears to be encased by the tumour. 3 lymph nodes are found at the fatty tissue attached. Blocks are taken as follows - (A) Gastric remnant margin and duodenal margin, 2 tissue blocks. (B) Pancreatic margin, 1 tissue block. Common bile duct margin, 1 tissue block. (C) to (H) Tumour, 6 tissue blocks with inclusion of the portal vein. (I) 3 tissue blocks from the lymph nodes. Figure (4) shows the submitted specimen. Figure (5) shows its cut surface.

MICROSCOPIC EXAMINATION:

1to4) Section from the tumour in the pancreas shows infiltration by adenocarcinoma. The tumour cells are arranged in irregular complex neoplastic glandular structure infiltrating fibroblastic stroma. The tumour cells show mild to moderate cellular atypia. Some of the tumour cells possess cytoplasmic mucin. Lymphovascular permeation is not seen in the sampled tissue blocks. There is tumour infiltration into the wall of the portal vein included in the specimen. There is tumour extension into the peripancreatic soft tissue. There is also focal tumour infiltration into the muscularis propria of the duodenal wall. The submucosa and the mucosa of the duodenum is not infiltrated. The tumour is very close to the circumferential adventitial resection margin. It measures <0.01 cm away from it. The common bile duct resection margin submitted in specimen (1) shows no tumour involvement. The frozen section of the pancreatic resection margin shows dysplasia in the bile duct. A tiny focus of perineural infiltration by tumour cells, however, is noted in the deeper paraffin section. This area measures <0.1 cm in size and it is not seen in the frozen section. The further pancreatic duct resection margin submitted in specimen (3) shows no dysplasia present. The resection margin from the gastric remnant and the duodenal margin are clear. All the 4 lymph nodes included in the specimen show no tumour metastasis. The overall features are those of a well to moderately differentiated adenocarcinoma.

Figure 1

Figure 2

Figure 3

Date of report :　12/11/2010

jw

Approved signatory: ....

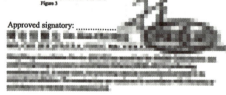

🎧 2010年11月10日病理报告示胰头癌，肿瘤侵及十二指肠、门静脉、神经组织等。 手术切缘距肿瘤组织小于0.01cm

医疗废物的危害

　　我们除了要提防辐射外，也要留意医疗废物所造成的危害。

　　医疗废物是医疗单位在医疗、预防、保健等相关过程和工作中产生的具有直接或间接感染性、病理性、损伤性、药物性、化学性的废物。

　　由于医疗废物具有全空间污染、急性传染和潜伏性污染等特征，其所含有的微生物的危害性是普通生活废物的几十、几百甚至上千倍，如处理不当，会成为医院感染和社会环境公害源，更严重则可成为疾病流行的源头。

　　医疗废物中含有不同程度的细菌、病毒和有害物质。而且废物中的有机物不仅滋生蚊蝇，造成疾病的传播，并且在腐败分解时释放出的氨气（NH_3）、硫化氢（H_2S）等恶臭气体会生成多种有害物质，污染大气，危害人体健康；同时医疗废物也是造成医院内交叉感染和空气污染的主要原因。

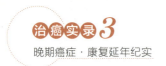
◇ **国内外医疗废物的危害现状**

感染性废物中的病原体可能通过呼吸系统、消化系统、肌肤上的切口、破损或刺破的伤口、黏膜等途径进入人体。另外，体液也是病原体的传播途径。所有面对医疗废物的个体都是高危人群，处于潜在的危险之中。

◇ **目前医疗废物的处理方式存在的危害**

常见的医疗废物处理方法有：焚烧、化学消毒、压力蒸汽消毒、辐射消毒、卫生填埋等，这些方法尚存在一定问题。如焚烧过程中会释放出几十种乃至上百种的金属"飞灰"和酸性气体，严重影响人体健康。医疗废物填埋处理需占据大量土地，会造成土地资源浪费及土壤污染。由于医疗废物有机物含量高，难分解，势必会造成环境、土地和地下水源受到二次污染，对人体健康构成危害。

晚期肺癌双肺转移肝转移，抗癌路上已 9 年

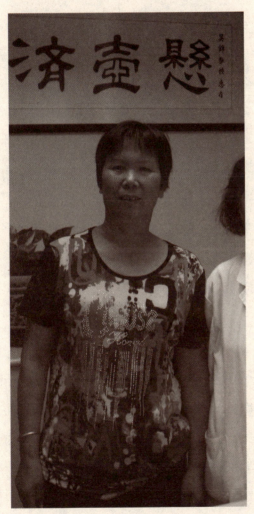

周女士于 2018 年 7 月来就诊时留影

周女士于 2009 年年初确诊晚期肺癌，经病理检验为恶性程度很高的低分化非小细胞肺癌，肿瘤很大，达 7.9cm。来诊前曾做化疗，但检查已属晚期，有双肺大量转移，大量淋巴转移，并有心包膜和胸壁的癌组织浸润。化疗没能控制肿瘤的快速生长和转移，她当时非常衰弱，全身无力，咳嗽频繁、胸痛气短。由于西医的治疗已全部做了，病

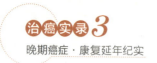
情仍继续发展和恶化，故于几个月后即前来进行生命修复中医药治疗。周女士服用中药后自感精神好转，症状改善，于是决定以中药做长期治疗。

补益脾肾，攻逐痰结。

治疗方案

(1) 常用中药：党参、茯苓、青礞石、山慈菇、川贝母、制甘遂、露蜂房、蛤蚧等。

(2) 散结丸、消瘤丸同时服用。

周女士自 2009 年开始一直坚持中医药治疗至 2015 年年底，近七年来自感一切都好，其间并多次复查，肿瘤明显缩小至消失。于是她放松治疗，逐渐不吃药了。但周女士于 2016 年 11 月又出现咳嗽，而且越来越重，至 2017 年 1 月检查有肿瘤复发，而且有肝转移。

周女士再次面对癌症复发、转移和生命危险。她很后悔停止了中医药的治疗，决定再下决心，认真用生命修复的中医药抗癌治癌。

经过治疗，患者病情渐趋稳定，咳嗽、疼痛等逐渐消失，至今周女士患晚期肺癌已有 9 年时间，她继续治疗，生活、工作均正常。

肺癌肝转移是晚期肺癌常见表现之一，治疗的难度较大。肺癌肝转移治疗的效果直接影响到患者的生命长短和治疗的成败。当前西医药治疗认为，肺癌肝转移需要在控制原发癌肿的同时控制转移，在改善晚期患者生活质量的同时最大程度延长生存期。一般肺癌肝转移治疗方法主要包括局部姑息性手术治疗和放化疗。但手术的选择应慎重，需考虑病情的发展和患者的承受能力。常见的治疗方法如下。

1.肺癌肝转移局部姑息性手术治疗

肺癌肝转移多发生在晚期，手术治疗的概率较小，且术后往往会出现严重的并发症及复发转移，因此多不采用手术治疗。

2.肺癌肝转移的放化疗

放化疗作为单一的局部疗法，是肺癌肝转移治疗的主要方法，常结合使用，治疗前需综合评定患者的身体情况，因为放化疗的副作用比较严重，有时甚至不得不终止治疗，影响治疗效果。

由上述可知，实际上目前西医针对肺癌肝转移没有很好的治疗方法，也很难控制疾病的发展。况且肺癌患者在有肝转移的同时，多伴有其他器官的转移，全身情况非常差，无法再进行手术、放化疗等。在这种情况下，我们仍有可靠的、有成熟经验的生命修复方法能够对患者进行有效的治疗。

附：患者相关检查报告

醫院 診斷及介入放射部
Department of Diagnostic & Interventional Radiology
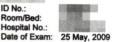
HOSPITAL

Name: CHAU,
Sex/Age/DOB: F/49/15-Jul-1959
Ref.Dr.:
Exam ID.:

ID No.:
Room/Bed:
Hospital No.:
Date of Exam: 25 May, 2009

CT SCAN OF THORAX WITH AND WITHOUT CONTRAST

Clinical data:
Chronic cough.

Technique:
One AP scout. 5 mm thick slices obtained at 5 mm intervals through the thorax with and without contrast (Ultravist).

Findings:
Malignant looking mass lesion measuring 6.1x5.4x7.9cm is noted in the lingula of L upper lobe. Medially, it is seen invading into the pericardium (se 301, image 309). Laterally, it is seen abutting the chest wall. Posteriorly, it is seen abutting the L oblique fissure which is itself irregular in some region with tongue of opacity extending into the L lower lobe. Findings are suggestive of tumoral invasion across the L oblique fissure.

Rest of the lungs are clear. No mass lesion is noted. No bronchiectasis is seen. No pleural or pericardial effusion is seen.

Enlarged L hilar lymph node is noted (Se 301, image 217). Prominent lymph node is seen in the aortopulmonary window (Se 301, image 165). Shotty lymph nodes are seen in the rest of the mediastinum (pretracheal, R, L paratracheal, precarinal and prevascular).

Imaged portion of liver and adrenals appear unremarkable. Enlarged lymph nodes are seen in the L anterior costophrenic sulcus (Se 301, image 386).

Impression:
1. Malignant looking mass lesion (6.1x5.4x7.9cm) in lingula of L upper lobe, invading into the pericardium and across the L oblique fissure into the L lower lobe. It is closely abutting the chest wall. Tissue diagnosis is suggested for further assessment.
2. Lymphadenopathy in L hilar region and L anterior costophrenic sulcus. Prominent aortopulmonary window lymph node. Shotty mediastinal lymph nodes.

Dr

-1-

🎧 2009 年 5 月 25 日检查报告示肺肿瘤 7.9cm，并侵入心包，紧贴胸壁等，而且肺门、主肺动脉窗、纵隔、气管周围等多处可见淋巴转移病灶

HONG KONG SANATORIUM & HOSPITAL

Histopathology Laboratory

PATIENT 'S NAME		DATE RECEIVED		PATHOLOGY NO.	COPY:
周 ■ CHAU ■ ■		26/05/2009		■ ■ ■	DR.
I. D. NO.	SEX F	AGE 49 Y			
■ ■	HOSPITAL NO. ■ ■	CLASS ■ ■		PREVIOUS PATH. NO. ■ ■	

UNDER CARE OF DR.	Dr. ■ ■ / Dr. Li Ka Wah
DOCTOR'S ADDRESS	■ ■ Hospital.
CLINICAL PROCEDURE	Core biopsies left lingular lung mass.
CLINICAL SUMMARY	Cough and haemoptysis two months. CT scan - mass in left lingular segment / left lower lobe invading pericardium. ? Carcinoma.
FROZEN SECTION DIAGNOSIS (if any)	Severe inflammation - Focal mild atypia. Please await paraffin.
PATHOLOGICAL DIAGNOSIS	Left lung (core biopsies) - Poorly differentiated non-small cell carcinoma. - Favour lymphoepithelioma-like carcinoma. - Pending EBV ISH and EGFR gene mutation analysis.

REPORT

Macroscopic examination:

(1) "Left lung biopsy" - A greyish to tan-coloured core 1.6 cm. long and 0.1 cm. in diameter.

(2) "Left lung biopsy" - Five tan-coloured cores, largest 1.8 cm. and 0.5 cm. long, each 0.1 cm. in diameter.

Microscopic examination:

(1) Paraffin section confirms the frozen section appearances and shows cores of fibrotic lung tissue with dense chronic inflammatory infiltration including many small lymphocytes. Occasional clusters of crushed atypical large cells are seen suspicious but not diagnostic of carcinoma.

(2) Cores of lung tissue show extensive infiltration by poorly defined nests of large cohesive malignant epithelial cells, with many admixed small lymphocytes and associated acute-on-chronic inflammatory infiltration as well as fibrosis. The lesional cells show focal syncytial morphology with hyperchromatic pleomorphic nuclei, focally prominent central nucleoli and moderate amounts of amphophilic cytoplasm. The appearances are a poorly differentiated non-small cell carcinoma, perhaps most likely lymphoepithelioma-like carcinoma. A further report will follow confirmatory EBV in-situ hybridization studies, as well as EGFR gene mutation analysis.

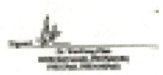

Date Reported: 27/05/2009

❶ 2009 年 5 月 26 日病理报告示低分化非小细胞癌

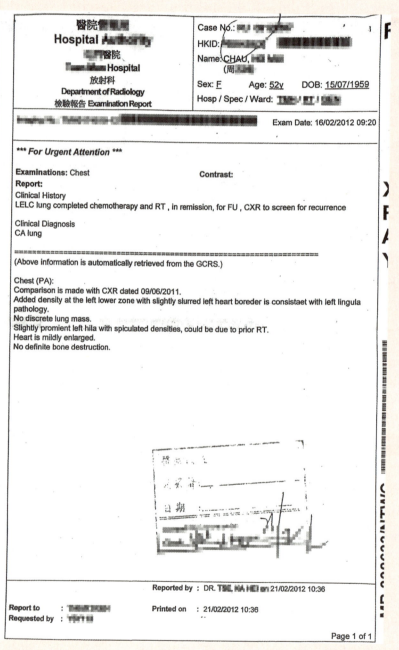

醫院 Hospital Authority
醫院
Hospital
放射科
Department of Radiology
檢驗報告 Examination Report

Case No.:
HKID:
Name: CHAU,
(周
Sex: F   Age: 52y   DOB: 15/07/1959
Hosp / Spec / Ward:

Exam Date: 16/02/2012 09:20

*** For Urgent Attention ***

Examinations: Chest   **Contrast:**

Report:
Clinical History
LELC lung completed chemotherapy and RT , in remission, for FU , CXR to screen for recurrence

Clinical Diagnosis
CA lung

===
(Above information is automatically retrieved from the GCRS.)

Chest (PA):
Comparison is made with CXR dated 09/06/2011.
Added density at the left lower zone with slightly slurred left heart boreder is consistaet with left lingula pathology.
No discrete lung mass.
Slightly promient left hila with spiculated densities, could be due to prior RT.
Heart is mildly enlarged.
No definite bone destruction.

Reported by : DR. TSE, NA HEI on 21/02/2012 10:36

Report to   :
Requested by :   Printed on   : 21/02/2012 10:36

Page 1 of 1

❶ 2012 年检查报告显示肺部无肿瘤生长

136

食品添加剂的危害

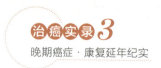
◇ 什么是食品添加剂

常见的食品添加剂有防腐剂、抗氧化剂、漂白剂、酸味剂、凝固剂、疏松剂、增稠剂、甜味剂、着色剂、乳化剂、品质改良剂、增味剂等。

按常用食品添加剂的功能可以将其归纳为以下几类。

(1) 为改善品质而加入的色素、香料、漂白剂、增味剂、甜味剂、膨松剂等。

(2) 为防止食品腐败变质而加入的抗氧化剂和防腐剂等。

(3) 为便于加工而加入的稳定剂、乳化剂、消泡剂等。

(4) 为增加食品营养价值而加入的营养强化剂，如维生素、微量元素等。

◇ 防腐剂

日常生活中，从调味品中的酱油、果酱到各类糕点、饮料及各种加工食物、包装食物中都少不了添加防腐剂。防腐剂可以防止食物腐败变质，抑制微生物生长，有时也可以防止食物中毒之类问题的产生。这些无疑是有益于消费者健康与安全的。

防腐剂都是由人工合成的，常见的有苯甲酸、苯甲酸钠、山梨酸、山梨酸钾等。

超标使用防腐剂会对人体造成一定伤害，轻则会引起流口水、腹泻、肚痛、心搏加快等症状，重则会对胃、肝、肾造成严重危害，更会增加癌症的罹患率。

◇ 色素

色素并非违法添加物，在食品中添加色素也不是现代人才发明的。在中国古代，人们就知道利用红曲色素来制造红酒。食用色素只要在国家许可的范围和标准内使用（婴幼儿食品中是严禁使用任何人工合成色素的）就不会对健康造成危害。但是，总是有一些不法商贩为了追逐利润而过量添加色素。数年前爆发的"苏丹红事件"，其恶劣的影响使大众对原本名声就不太好的色素更加产生了怀疑。当然，苏丹红其实是一种工业染料而非可食用色素。

商家为了增加消费者的食欲，会使用人工合成的色素添加剂。常见的有苋菜红、胭脂红、柠檬黄、日落黄、焦糖色素等人工合成色素。消费者在选择食品时，切记不要被那艳丽的外衣所迷惑，应避免购买过分鲜艳的食品。

人工色素是从煤焦油中提炼出来的。过量使用人工色素会加速孩子体内锌元素的流失，结果可能会出现多动症、情绪烦躁、生长发育迟缓、智力发育迟缓、异食癖等，成年男性则会发生生殖障碍，因为精子的合成需要锌。

天然色素从动、植物中提取是安全的食用色素，但因其来源少、价格高，使用并不广泛。

◇ 膨松剂

面包、馒头、油条、饼干等许多糕点都会使用膨松剂。专

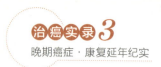

家分析了市场上的膨化食品、一些油炸制品、发酵面制品及部分糖果和巧克力制品等，发现常用的膨松剂有碳酸氢钠（$NaHCO_3$，俗称苏打粉）、碳酸氢铵（NH_4HCO_3，俗称臭粉）、复合膨松剂等。

膨松剂食品内都存在铝超标的问题。铝不是人体必需的微量元素，而是有害健康的，它会干扰细胞和器官的正常代谢，造成神经系统病变，如记忆力衰退、脑损伤、智力下降、视觉障碍、运动失调甚至痴呆等。

◇ 增稠剂

增稠剂是一类亲水性的高分子化合物，可以起到增稠的效果。如羧甲基纤维素钠、海藻酸钠、果胶、卡拉胶、阿拉伯胶、黄原胶、明胶、琼脂等。

◇ 酸味调节剂

为制造食品酸酸甜甜的口感，食品制造商会加入柠檬酸、酒石酸、乳酸、苹果酸等酸味调节剂在加工食品中。

◇ 乳化剂

乳化剂常见于一些乳制品或者乳类饮料，常用的有单硬脂酸甘油酯等。

◇ 反式脂肪酸

各种各样添加剂调制出来的"美味"食品中都有很多反式脂肪酸的存在。反式脂肪酸是人体难以消化处理的脂肪，一吃入肚就可能危害健康。反式脂肪酸在自然食品中含量很少，人们平时食用的含有反式脂肪酸的食品基本上来自含有人造奶油的食品。为增加货架期和产品稳定性而添加氢化油的产品中都可以发现反式脂肪酸，包括人造黄油特别是软性人造黄油、薄脆饼干、焙烤食品、谷类食品、面包和快餐中的油炸食品如炸薯条、炸鱼、洋葱圈等。

反式脂肪酸的名称不一，一般都在商品包装上标注为"氢化植物油""植物起酥油""人造黄油""人造奶油""人造牛油""植物奶油""马芝连""乳玛琳""植脂末"等。据了解在同一家超市里，95 种饼干里有 36 种、51 种蛋糕点心里有 19 种、全部 16 种咖啡伴侣以及 31 种麦片里有 22 种都含有反式脂肪酸。面包、糖果、冰淇淋、速冻汤圆等也不能"幸免"。而且许多著名品牌的产品都含有这些成分。

中国疾病预防控制中心营养与食品安全所联合北京市营养

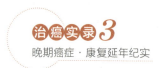
源研究所对市面上的 21 种点心进行了调查，分析了其中反式脂肪酸的含量。结果发现：超过 30% 的此类点心反式脂肪酸含量都在 2% 以上！而世界卫生组织建议反式脂肪酸每日每人摄入量不要超过总能量的 1%，即大约每天不超过 2 克。

如果每天吃 3 个这样的糕饼点心，反式脂肪酸摄入就极易超标。而摄入过多的反式脂肪酸会损伤肝脏、降低记忆力；在腹部堆积而造成发胖，脂肪堆积；增加血液黏稠度，容易形成血栓；导致一些慢性病的发展，如高血压、高血脂、高胆固醇、心脑血管病、糖尿病、癌症等。还会影响胎儿、婴儿和青少年的生长发育，影响儿童的智力发育，增加中年人患心脑血管疾病、糖尿病的风险，也会影响生育能力，加速老年人认知功能衰退，增加老年痴呆症发生的风险。

◇ **甜味剂**

甜味剂是赋予食品以甜味的添加剂，常用的有：阿斯巴甜、糖精钠（习惯上称的糖精）、环己基氨基磺酸钠（甜蜜素）、麦芽糖醇、山梨糖醇、木糖醇等。因为它们的代谢不受胰岛素控制，不会升高血糖。

1. 糖精

糖精是最古老的人工甜味剂，一百年前就已经被使用在食物或药品上。因为糖精在体内不会转化为葡萄糖且能快速吸收排出体外，不会增加热量，于是受到糖尿病患者和节食者的欢迎。20世纪60年代研究发现，糖精可能导致膀胱癌，于是越来越多的食品中改用阿斯巴甜（Aspartame, 简称APM）。

2. 阿斯巴甜（代糖，APM）

据报道，全球有超过10亿人口摄取含有阿斯巴甜的饮食，并相信这种成分不具危险性，但是美国食品及药物管理局在2010年左右接获的不良反应投诉中，有大量是由阿斯巴甜引起的。

阿斯巴甜是一种合成化学物质，在人体胃肠道酶作用下可分解为大约含有50%苯丙氨酸、40%天冬氨酸及10%甲醇。食物、饮料、糖果、口香糖、维生素、健康补充品甚至处方药物等都含有APM。

APM所含的三种成分各有其危险性，而且每一种都会造成许多副作用及危害健康的问题。其所含成分如下。

• 苯丙氨酸（Phenylalanine）：血液中大量的苯丙氨酸可能会集中在大脑的某些部位，对幼儿及胎儿特别有害。苯丙氨酸能导致脑部永久伤害甚至死亡，尤其是在大量进食或怀孕期间。

• 天冬氨酸（Aspartic acid）：天冬氨酸被认为是一种神经兴奋毒素，也就是说这种成分会过度刺激某些神经直到神经死亡。如同硝酸盐及味精，天冬氨酸可造成体内氨基酸失衡并干扰大脑神经递质代谢。

• 甲醇（Methanol）：阿斯巴甜最大的危害是甲醇（木醇），甲醇会循环至全身（包括大脑、肌肉、脂肪及神经组织），接着代谢成为甲醛。甲醇是一种危险的神经毒素，也是已知的致癌物质，可能造成视网膜受损、致盲，干扰DNA并导致先天缺陷。

阿斯巴甜的不良反应包括晕眩、头痛、行为改变、幻觉、忧郁、恶心、麻痹、肌肉痉挛、体重增加、皮疹、疲劳、易怒、失眠、视力问题、丧失听觉、心悸、呼吸困难、焦虑、口齿不清、失去味觉、耳鸣、晕眩、丧失记忆及关节疼痛等，与纤维肌痛及多重硬化症的症状相似。同时，许多疾病也会因为摄取阿斯巴甜而更为恶化，包括慢性疲劳症候群、大脑肿瘤、癫痫、帕金森病、阿尔茨海默症、精神发育迟缓及糖尿病等。

有关多项研究已经指出，阿斯巴甜可导致癌症、淋巴瘤、白血病、器官损害、癌细胞转移、神经受损、痉挛及早死等病症。还有研究指出，苯丙氨酸会集中在胎盘，导致胎儿精神发育迟缓。同时，怀孕女性血液中的苯丙氨酸也会促使其体内的免疫系统将胎儿视为外来物质而将其摧毁，导致流产。

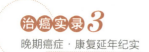
13

晚期前列腺癌已 9 年，现今 81 岁不言老

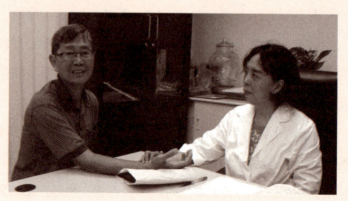

🎙 黄先生于 2018 年 7 月来中心合影留念

　　黄先生81岁了，健康快乐，红光满面，常来中心调理身体，但谁也看不出他曾是晚期癌症患者。黄先生于2009年72岁时，常发生尿急，排尿困难，并越来越严重，此后又出现髋骨、腰背等全身疼痛和骨痛，于是到医院就诊。当时疼痛严重，夜晚时常痛醒，不能小便，需要医院导尿，不能进食，非常虚弱。因全身疼痛做全身CT检查，发现有前列腺癌。又经病理组织学检查证实，有全身多发性的骨转移。当时癌病已属晚期，在右侧髋骨、腰椎、肋骨等多处又发生骨转移，无法进行手术，医生讲只能对症治疗，没有很好的办法。黄先生不想就此了结，经多方打听，来进行生命修复的中医药治疗。他全身无力，行动困难，腰背疼痛严重，排尿困难。

 治疗原则

补肾益气，涤痰化毒。

治疗方案

(1) 常用中药：人参、茯苓、白术、仙灵脾、肉苁蓉、炮山甲、青礞石、莪术、重楼、贝母等。

(2) 消瘤丸同时服用。

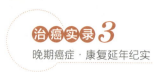

经辨证他的病情为本虚标实，本虚以肾气亏虚、脾气亏虚为主，标实以气滞、痰毒为主。黄先生在治疗中逐渐改善进食，体重增加，精神、气色改善，不断进步。

黄先生于 2010 年 8 月的检查报告显示前列腺癌多发骨转移，于 2014 年 6 月的检查报告显示多发骨转移全部消失，在运用生命修复的 4 年左右中医药治疗过程中，他并没有用过化疗、放疗或激素治疗。由发现癌症至今，9 年过去了，他感到身体比年轻时更好，并常说有信心更加长寿。

前列腺癌发病隐蔽，不易早期诊断，多数患者发现时已属晚期，而且几乎都会发展为激素非依赖型的晚期前列腺癌（HRPC），这是现代医学的治疗难点。尤其 HRPC 患者，现代医学目前仍缺乏有效的治疗方法。据报道，HRPC 患者的中位生存期在 10 ~ 52 周，现代医学研究显示目前的治疗方案并不能明显延长生存期，美国每年大约有 4.2 万例 HRPC 患者死亡。

生命修复中医药治疗的精髓在于攻补兼施，整体论治，辅助正气。首先控制癌细胞的迅猛发展势头，再进一步缩小肿瘤，控制并治疗转移病灶。中医古籍《医学入门·溺血》论述："暴热实热利之宜，虚损房劳兼日久，滋阴补肾更无疑。"久病虚损，治疗应扶正补虚；清代程钟龄称："脏腑、筋络、肌肉之间，本无此物而忽有之，必为消散，乃得其平。"必须要有祛邪的方法，才能使癌肿消散。

附：患者相关检查报告

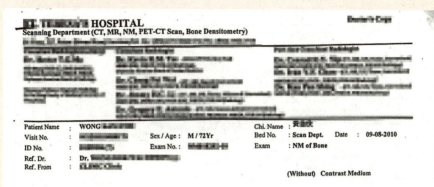

HOSPITAL
Scanning Department (CT, MR, NM, PET-CT Scan, Bone Densitometry)

Patient Name	: WONG				Chi. Name	: 黄	
Visit No.	:	Sex / Age :	M / 72Yr		Bed No.	: Scan Dept.	Date : 09-08-2010
ID No.	:	Exam No. :			Exam	: NM of Bone	
Ref. Dr.	: Dr.						
Ref. From	:						

(Without) Contrast Medium

Clinical Information / History:

Prostate biopsy confirmed Ca prostate. PSA = 92.

Radiological Report:

Whole body bone scan was performed after the intravenous injection of 25 mCi Tc-99m MDP.

FINDINGS :

Planar and SPECT images of the skeleton demonstrate intense abnormal uptake at the inferior aspect of the right ilium. This is most consistent with bone metastasis. No disease activity is demonstrated in other areas in the bony pelvis. Abnormal uptake is also demonstrated at L3 vertebral body. Again, this is most consistent with bone metastasis. No significant abnormality is demonstrated in other vertebra levels. Mild focal uptake is also demonstrated at the posterior aspect of the left 9th rib. This may represent subradiographic bone injury or early metastasis. The sternum, clavicles and scapulae are normal. No significant abnormality is present in the skull and extremities.

IMPRESSION :

Abnormal uptake is present at L3 and the right ilium. These are most consistent with bone metastases. Mild focal uptake at the 9th rib may represent subclinical rib injury or early metastasis.

Thank you for your referral.

				(DDMM) (HHMM)		
NO. OF FILMS	0	14" x 17"			REPORT & FILMS SENT OUT :	
NO. OF COLOR PRINT	5	NO. OF CDR 1	'WET' FILMS: SENT		09-08-2010	PM DHL
Remark :			RETURNED			

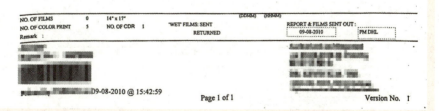

09-08-2010 @ 15:42:59   Page 1 of 1   Version No. 1

❶ 2010 年 8 月 9 日检查报告显示前列腺癌多发骨转移

醫院 ▓▓▓	Case No.: ▓▓▓▓	R
Hospital ▓▓▓▓	HKID: ▓▓▓▓▓▓	
▓▓▓▓ 醫院	Name: WONG, ▓▓▓▓	
▓▓▓ Hospital	（黄 ▓▓）	
影像及介入放射科	Sex: M Age: 76y DOB: 1938	
Department of Imaging and Interventional Radiology (DIIR)	Hosp / Spec / Ward: ▓▓▓ ▓▓▓ ▓▓▓	
檢驗報告Examination Report		

▓▓▓▓▓▓▓ ▓▓▓▓▓▓▓ ▓▓▓▓▓▓▓▓▓▓▓▓   Reg. Date: 25-Jun-2014 10:50

N
M

Procedure: Bone WB MDP

Pharmaceutical: Tc99m MDP I.V 20.00 mCi

Clinical Information (from referring clinician):
ca prostate with bil orchidectomy done in 2010 Complaint of vague back pain at thorcic level

Diagnosis (from referring clinician):
ca prostate

Report:

BONE SCAN

PROCEDURE
mCi Tc-99m MDP i.v.
Static planar imaging of the wholebody skeleton.

FINDINGS
MDP biodistribution is within normal limits.
Focal uptake is present in the left shoulder acromioclavicular joint. Corresponding XRs shows mild osteoarthrosis.

No other suspicious uptake is present.

IMPRESSION
1. No evidence of bony metastases.
2. Focal uptake in left AC joint is likely related to underlying degenerative change.lkl126

Additional Information

Accession no.: ▓▓▓▓▓▓▓▓▓   **Modality:** XRAY   **Reg. Date:** 25-Jun-2014 15:04

Procedure: Shoulder

Requested by: ILLEGIBLE

| Reported by : DR. ▓▓▓▓▓▓▓ ▓▓▓ 25-Jun-2014 16:35 |
| Report to : ▓▓▓▓▓▓▓ |
| Requested by : ▓▓▓▓▓▓▓   Generated on : 25-Jun-2014 16:35 |

Page 1 of 1

♬ 2014 年 6 月 25 日检查报告显示多发骨转移消失

食肉过多有何不良影响

　　不同疾病的统计资料显示，肉类消耗得多的地区，罹患心脏病、癌症等疾病的比率不断地增高，而素食为主的地区，罹病的比率就低得多。

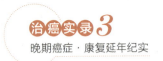

◇ 动物疾病

在现代的饲养过程中，动物已完全脱离正常的生长环境，被逼生长在窄小的、恶劣的、非自然的人工环境中，使得动物从初生开始就没有见过阳光。为适宜生存，它们的身体就开始对抗这种非自然的生活并分泌各种不正常的有害物质，这种环境也改变了它们的自然习性，使之更易患各种疾病。

动物体内发生的疾病、肿瘤及生长环境中的寄生虫、细菌、病毒等并不是全部都能检测出来或者并不是全部要求检测出来的。

据很多报道显示，动物有病的部分切掉之后，剩余部分还是会拿去卖掉。甚至有些商家会将有病的切除部分制成罐头、香肠等。

◇ 药物残留毒素

在饲养场内，为降低死亡、缩短养殖过程，动物会被注射各种药物，如抗生素、生长激素、开胃药、镇静剂、瘦肉精、多肉精等人创造出来的各类不同的有害化学物质，也大量给予各种人造饲料、强化饲料等非正常饲料及各式各样的不适当添加剂，动物吃进的各种不洁、有毒有害物质会大量残留于动物体内成为毒素，对人体健康造成严重危害。

◇ 屠宰产生毒素

　　动物被杀之前的恐惧以及被杀之中的痛苦，使身体的内分泌、神经、血液等各个系统迅速产生了极大的变化，并在应激状态下释放出大量的各种各样的有害物质而使得整体都被毒化了。根据有关检测，动物体中有大量毒素，包括尿酸及其他各种有毒的排泄物都进入了血液与身体组织之内。

　　正如我们在恐惧、愤怒、紧张之中会得病，各种动物无异于人类，它们在危险的情况中内分泌等功能同样会产生极大的化学变化。动物血液中的激素如肾上腺素等大量分泌，使得其分泌系统发生彻底地改变。大量的毒素、激素等留在肉内会进一步毒化人们的身体组织。动物尸体的肉中含有大量有毒的血液与代谢中的排泄物和化学毒素。

　　当动物死亡后，尸体中的蛋白质就会凝结并且发生自我分解。很快地，一种名为"尸毒"的变性物质就形成了。由于在死亡后就会立刻释放出这些毒素，各种肉、鱼类以及蛋类会很快地分解、腐败。冷藏或加防腐剂只能降低腐败的速度，并不能完全停止腐败。从动物被屠杀到放到餐桌上烹饪完毕，这期间经历了很多时间和各种处理过程，当然已经腐坏到相当严重的程度了。

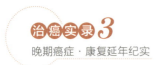
◇ **生物链污染**

在自然界有一条长长的食物链：植物吸收阳光、空气、水
→动物吃植物→大动物或人类吃小动物。

当今，环境污染问题日趋严重，农田、牧场和水域都被污
染，这些污染物包括化肥、农药、各种有机和无机的化合物及
工业污染等，动物通过吃植物而使这些有害物质在体内大量储
存。譬如农田、鱼塘里喷洒 DDT 作为除虫剂，这是一种强烈的
毒药，足以导致癌症、不孕或严重的肝病等。DDT 以及其他类
似的杀虫剂，会保存在动物及鱼类脂肪内，并且一旦储存便很
难破坏。当牛吃草或饲料时，不论它们吃下了哪种杀虫剂，大
部分都会残存在它们体内，当人们吃肉时，就把 DDT 以及其他
累积在动物身体内的毒素都吃进了体内。由于吃的是食物链末
端的食物，所以人类就变成有毒高浓度杀虫剂的最后吸收者。
据调查，某池塘养殖的各种鱼通过吃水中的藻类和浮游生物等，
使鱼体内的杀虫剂"六六六"的浓度比池塘水中的含量高十几
倍到几十倍。

◇ **烹调及储存产生的危害**

肉类脂肪在烹饪加热至高温时会形成甲基胆蒽
（Methylcholanthrene）、苯并芘（Benzopyrene）等有害物质，增加
患者癌的概率。

肉存放时，很快就会自然腐败变成病态的青灰色。于是肉商会在肉里非法加入硝酸盐、亚硝酸盐或其他防腐剂，这些东西使肉类呈现出鲜红色。冻肉在制作过程中同样加入了各种防腐剂、添加剂、矫味剂等有害物质。

 病案 14

晚期睾丸癌双肺转移，正常生活已 8 年

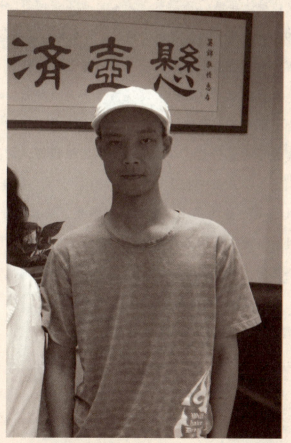

洪先生于 2018 年 5 月来研究中心留影

洪先生2010年下半年常有咳嗽，多痰，阴部肿胀不适，那时他24岁，每日忙忙碌碌，早起上班，晚饭后在家里不停地玩游戏机，熬夜不睡觉是常事。他认为只是缺少睡眠，所以精力不足，白天无力嗜睡，双腿发沉。很长时间以来也容易感冒，他认为这大概是感冒时间较长，总也没有彻底清除感冒的结果。这样拖了大半年之后，他认为感冒还没有好，又出现了下肢肿胀，阴部肿胀更加明显。他的母亲多次问他有哪里不舒服，并反复要求他晚上早睡，不要熬夜，他总也不当回事。洪先生的父亲在59岁时就患了癌症并已离世了，母亲特别紧张他的身体。有一天他让母亲去给买一双大一号码的鞋，因为鞋子太小穿不进去。母亲仔细看看他的脚，发现两只脚是很肿胀，感到有问题，于是立即带他去医院，结果于2011年6月发现睾丸癌并有双肺及胸腔等大量转移。洪先生的妈妈泪流满面，求医生救救自己的儿子。于是洪先生于2011年7月做手术切除睾丸肿瘤，以后又做了高剂量的化疗，当时病情危重，胸痛、呼吸困难、腹痛，西医认为该做的治疗都做了，已无法可医，医院估计他只有几个月的生命。经多方打听，洪先生的妈妈带他来求治于生命修复的中医药治疗。

当时他骨瘦如柴，自己不能行走，25岁的年轻人，却需要一手拄着拐杖，另一手扶在母亲的肩上，才能够移动一下。气短，气急，呼吸困难，胸痛。

患者病性属本虚标实，阴虚毒聚，经脉壅滞，瘀毒结聚，以补正滋补肝肾，化瘀通络，解毒抗癌。

治疗原则

滋补肝肾，解毒化瘀。

治疗方案

(1) 菟丝子、杜仲、肉苁蓉、海藻、昆布、半枝莲、皂角刺、川芎、莪术、三棱等。

(2) 消瘤丸同时服用。

就这样，洪先生开始了生命修复的中医药治疗。每天由他的母亲帮他看时间，按时服药，也配合做一些辅助治疗如针灸和敷中药。日子一天天过去，他的病情慢慢好转，脸上渐渐有了红润的颜色，体重增加。几个月后不再需要拐杖，以后逐渐行走、跑步自如，生活正常，已2年多不能工作的他又可以去上班了，恢复了正常的工作。

如今8年过去了，他的生活和工作正常。虽然肺部仍有残留少许转移病灶，但是并没有影响到正常的生活，我们大家也在一起努力，争取早日帮他全面消除残余病灶。

附：患者相关检查报告

Hospital [illegible]

[illegible] Park [illegible]

HKID: [illegible]

Name: HUNG, [illegible]

DOB: 19/02/1986

Sex: M   Age: 25y

Case No.	[illegible]	Record No.	[illegible]	Last Report Date	02/07/2011
Test Name	[illegible]	Site	[illegible]		

Final Report   08/07/2011

Clinical History
Carcinoma of right testis with lung secondaries.

Gross Examination
A orchidectomy specimen that weighed 157 g. The testis had been previously bisected open and measured 7 cm x 4.5 cm x 4.0 cm. The tunica albuginea surface was smooth. The spermatic cord measured 9 cm long with diameter of 1 cm. Cut surfaces of the testis showed a circumscribed lobulated tumour that measured 6.8 cm x 3.8 cm x 3.5 cm with variegated appearance containing solid whitish nodular areas, haemorrhagic, necrotic and cystic foci. A compressed rim of tan brown testicular parenchyma that measured up to 7 mm thick was present in the periphery. The tumour appeared intratesticular with no involvement of the tunica. The epididymis measured 3 cm x 2 cm x 1 cm and was unremarkable.

Total 17 Blocks.
(A1-A11, A14-A16) Tumour including residual testis.
(A12) Spermatic cord.
(A13) Spermatic cord resection margin.
(A17) Epididymis.

Microscopic Examination
The tumour shows a mixed germ cell tumour featuring haphazard mixture of mostly teratoma (60%), embryonal carcinoma (35%) components with small foci of choriocarcinoma (5%). The teratoma shows mature and immature elements including squamous epithelium, smooth muscle and cartilage, gastrointestinal epithelium and blastemal tissue. There are patchy intermixed areas of embryonal carcinoma displaying solid and anastomosing glandular foci of large, syncytial and polygonal cells (CD30+) containing enlarged hyperchromatic nuclei, coarse chromatin, macronucleoli and moderate amount of amphophilic cytoplasm. Frequent mitotic activities and necrosis are present. Foci of choriocarcinoma are noted (A10 & A16) and feature giant syncytiotrophoblasts (beta-HCG+) intermingled with cytotrophoblasts associated with prominent areas of haemorrhage. Lymphovascular permeation is observed but no tunica albuginea invasion is seen. Focal intratubular germ cell neoplasia (ITGCN) (OCT3/4+) is present in the residual atrophic seminiferous tubules. The rete testis, epididymis, the spermatic cord and its resection margin are unremarkable.

Diagnosis
TESTIS, right, orchidectomy
- MIXED GERM CELL TUMOUR containing TERATOMA, EMBRYONAL CARCINOMA and CHORIOCARCINOMA components;
- INTRATUBULAR GERM CELL NEOPLASIA.

⋒ 2011 年 7 月 2 日病理报告示睾丸生殖细胞癌、胚胎癌

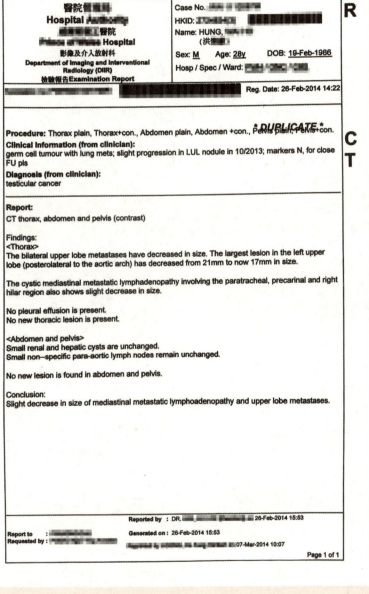

医院 〓〓〓〓
Hospital 〓〓〓〓
〓〓〓〓 医院
〓〓〓〓〓〓 **Hospital**
影像及介入放射科
Department of Imaging and Interventional Radiology (DIIR)
检验报告 **Examination Report**

Case No.
HKID:
Name: HUNG,
(洪〓〓)
Sex: **M**   Age: **28y**   DOB: **19-Feb-1986**
Hosp / Spec / Ward:

Reg. Date: 26-Feb-2014 14:22

R

C T

DUPLICATE

Procedure: Thorax plain, Thorax+con., Abdomen plain, Abdomen +con., Pelvis plain, Pelvis+con.
Clinical Information (from clinician):
germ cell tumour with lung mets; slight progression in LUL nodule in 10/2013; markers N, for close FU pls
Diagnosis (from clinician):
testicular cancer

Report:
CT thorax, abdomen and pelvis (contrast)

Findings:
<Thorax>
The bilateral upper lobe metastases have decreased in size. The largest lesion in the left upper lobe (posterolateral to the aortic arch) has decreased from 21mm to now 17mm in size.

The cystic mediastinal metastatic lymphadenopathy involving the paratracheal, precarinal and right hilar region also shows slight decrease in size.

No pleural effusion is present.
No new thoracic lesion is present.

<Abdomen and pelvis>
Small renal and hepatic cysts are unchanged.
Small non—specific para-aortic lymph nodes remain unchanged.

No new lesion is found in abdomen and pelvis.

Conclusion:
Slight decrease in size of mediastinal metastatic lymphoadenopathy and upper lobe metastases.

Reported by : DR.   26-Feb-2014 15:53

Report to   :
Requested by :

Generated on : 26-Feb-2014 15:53

                                                           07-Mar-2014 10:07

Page 1 of 1

🎧 2014 年 2 月 26 日检查报告示纵隔及肺部转移灶缩小

水的质量及转基因问题

◇ 饮用水的质量

为了保证卫生，现在全球大多数自来水都有经过氯消毒，潜伏在自来水中的罪魁祸首是三卤甲烷。自来水在净水场加氯消毒过程中，水中有机物（例如食物的渣滓和蜉蝣生物等）和氯相互反应会形成三卤甲烷，其主要的生成物包括三氯甲烷、二氯溴甲烷、三氯溴甲烷和三溴甲烷等氯化物。在用三氯甲烷对白鼠和狗进行的 9 项实验中，有 5 项证实其能引发肝癌或肾癌，其他 3 种氯化物也有一定的致癌性。随着水质的恶化，自来水中氯的投放量也与日俱增，间接扮演了制造致癌物的角色。

有研究表明，长期饮用氯消毒的自来水患膀胱癌的比率要比不长期饮用的人高出 35%，经常在游泳池里游泳的人患膀胱癌的概率比平常人高出 57%，造成这些现象的原因是氯在消毒的过程中会产生一些副产物。这些有毒物质会经过皮肤进入身体或经过呼吸进入体内，被人体吸收，大大提高了致癌的风险。

为了保证饮水健康，现在不少人都选择饮用矿泉水、蒸馏水，而事实上绝大多数人仍长期饮用自来水。在自来水生产的过程中会有各项保证安全的指标，将氯含量控制在人体饮用的限量范围之内，在一般情况下不会对身体造成严重危害。

饮用水以天然水为宜。自来水最好经过过滤以除去自来水消毒中含有的有害物质。

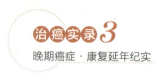

◇ 千滚水

千滚水就是在炉上沸腾了很长时间的水，还有电热水器中反复煮沸的水。这种水因煮过久，水中不挥发性物质如钙、镁等重金属成分和亚硝酸盐含量很高。久饮这种水会干扰人的胃肠功能，出现腹泻、腹胀；有毒的亚硝酸盐还会造成身体缺氧等严重问题。

◇ 蒸锅水

蒸锅水就是蒸馒头等剩锅水，多次反复使用的蒸锅水中亚硝酸盐浓度很高。常饮这种水或用这种水熬粥会引起亚硝酸盐中毒；水垢经常随水进入人体还会引起消化系统、神经系统、泌尿系统和造血系统病变，甚至引起早衰、癌症。

◇ 未煮沸的水

饮用未煮沸的水，患膀胱癌、直肠癌的可能性增加。当水温达到 100℃，卤代烃和氯仿这两种有害物质会随蒸气蒸发而大大减少，如继续沸腾 3min 则饮用安全。

◇ 转基因的问题

"转基因"是在不同生物类群之间转换基因，把完全不同科不同属甚至把跨物种生物的基因组合在一起，这种方式是正常的大自然界无法达到的，如将某种特别微生物基因转到主粮作物中，从而使得外来基因在自然界以不可控制方式传播。

基因改造技术将外来基因植入日常食物之中，如大豆、玉米、大米中，但基因改造食物在推出市场前都没有经过长远的安全评估，这就如同把人们当作白老鼠来做实验，有不可预测的风险。人类长期食用是否安全仍然成疑。转基因食品和转基因技术等毕竟是一种人类以往没有的、并无经验可以借鉴的新兴的技术，对其长远使用的安全性应当十分慎重。转基因农作物使用有毒性农药草甘膦等问题，我们已在相关章节说明。

15

晚期胆管癌肝转移，照料孙儿 12 年

古太太今年 81 岁了，在家看孙儿，忙里忙外，谁也看不出她是晚期癌症患者，而且她的癌症非常险恶，是俗称"癌王"的胆管癌。

十二年前，即 2006 年初，古太太常感右侧肋部、腹部疼痛，去医院检查后，医生讲有胆管炎，用消炎治疗，但疼痛还是越来越严重，于是她 2006 年 5 月份去医院做了胆囊切除手术，心想手术后应该很快就好了，但事与愿违，她的右侧腹部与肋部的疼痛没有因做

了手术而缓解，而是疼痛越来越加重，常常痛得不能睡觉，不能吃饭。无奈之下，儿子再次带她去医院做详细检查，先做了 CT 检查，于 2006 年 9 月诊断为胆管癌，并因拖延了时间，已经发生了肝脏的转移。医院认为她年岁大，又发生了肝转移，已经没有很好的治疗方法了。她疼痛越来越重，并出现越来越频

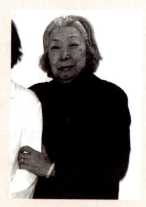

🔊 2018 年 6 月古太太生活正常愉快

繁的发热，还逐渐出现黄疸并很快加重。医生建议只能够做个支架暂时缓解一下，于是于 2006 年 12 月 30 日在胆管内放置一个支架。医生解释说，这样可使胆汁流出顺利一点，暂时缓解黄疸除此之外已无法可医。

万般无奈之下，她只能求助于生命修复治疗，古太太的儿子带她于 2007 年 1 月 9 日来就诊。

当时，她全身有严重黄疸，腹痛严重，不停呻吟。气短不续，下肢水肿。

治疗原则

解毒化湿，补中祛瘀。

治疗方案

(1) 常用中药：党参、田基黄、猪苓、鳖甲、延胡索、丹参、
海金沙、郁金、石见穿、白芍等。

(2) 消瘤丸同时服用。

治疗一年后她再次做了 CT 检查，肝内转移灶已全部消失（见后附检查报告）。如今 12 年过去了，古太太虽然已 81 岁高龄，但身体状况良好，承担着全部家务还照料着孙儿。她最终战胜了晚期胆管癌肝转移而完全康复，她也给予了许多患者极大的鼓舞和信心。发稿之际，我们再次打电话给她的儿子，询问患者目前状况，她儿子高兴地回答说，一切都很好，请我们放心，并再次表示谢意。

附：患者相关检查报告

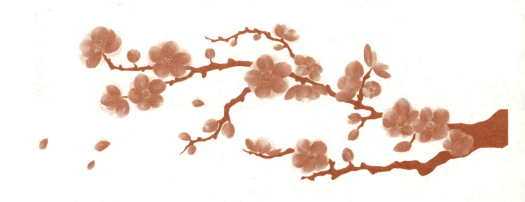

醫院	Case No.:
Hospital	HKID:
醫院	Name: CHIU,
Hospital	(趙
放射診斷部	Sex: **F** Age: **69y** DOB: **01/01/1937**
Radiology Department	Hosp / Spec / Ward:
檢驗報告 Examination Report	

R

Exam Date: 21/12/2006 9:15

* DUPLICATE *

C T

Examinations: Abdomen plain, Abdomen +con. **Contrast:**
Iomeron 400 (200ml) 80.00 ml

Report:
Contrast CT abdomen

History: Previous cholangitis and cholecystectomy. Obstructive jaundice

Technique: Pre and post contrast study of the abdomen according to the departmental protocol.

Findings:
Moderate dilatation of the intrahepatic biliary tree proximal to distal CBD narrowing. An internal biliary endoprosthesis noted in-situ bypassing the obstructive biliary system which is now filled with air and fluid.

Cholecystectomy with metallic surgical clips are noted.

A 2.5cm central necrotic tumor with rim enhancement noted segment 6 of liver compatible with metastasis. Small (<1cm) hypoenhancing mass at segment 8 and caudate lobe are too small to be accurately characterized. This could be a cyst or represent a metastatic deposit.

No focal pancreatic mass. The pancreatic ductal system is not dilated.

Spleen, adrenals and kidneys appear unremarkable.

Included lung bases and bony structures are clear.

No ascites or intra-abdominal adenopathy.

Atherosclerotic disease affecting the abdominal aorta with calcified plaques and small penetrating ulcers.

OPINIONS:
Malignant biliary obstruction due to cholangiocarcinoma with intrahepatic metastasis. The distal CBD stricture is bypassed by an internal biliary endoprosthesis. No regional adenopathy, ascites noted.

Nil adverse reaction.

THIS REPORT REQUIRES ATTENTION.

Reported by   21/12/2006 10:51

Report to   :
Requested by   :   Printed on   : 04/03/2008 14:20

Page 1 of 1

☊ 2006 年 12 月 21 日检查报告显示胆管癌胆管堵塞合并肝转移

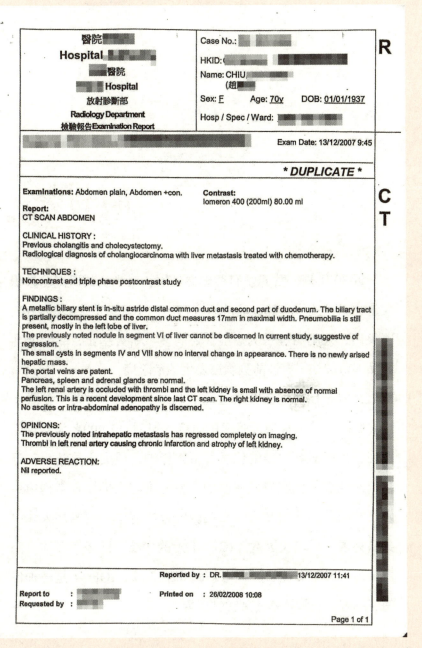

R

醫院 ▓▓▓	Case No.: ▓▓▓
Hospital ▓▓▓	HKID: ▓▓▓
▓▓▓ 醫院	Name: CHIU ▓▓▓
▓▓▓ **Hospital**	(超▓)
放射診斷部	Sex: <u>F</u> Age: <u>70y</u> DOB: <u>01/01/1937</u>
Radiology Department	Hosp / Spec / Ward: ▓▓▓
檢驗報告 Examination Report	

Exam Date: 13/12/2007 9:45

C T

* *DUPLICATE* *

Examinations: Abdomen plain, Abdomen +con.   **Contrast:**
Iomeron 400 (200ml) 80.00 ml

Report:
CT SCAN ABDOMEN

CLINICAL HISTORY :
Previous cholangitis and cholecystectomy.
Radiological diagnosis of cholangiocarcinoma with liver metastasis treated with chemotherapy.

TECHNIQUES :
Noncontrast and triple phase postcontrast study

FINDINGS :
A metallic biliary stent is in-situ astride distal common duct and second part of duodenum. The biliary tract is partially decompressed and the common duct measures 17mm in maximal width. Pneumobilia is still present, mostly in the left lobe of liver.
The previously noted nodule in segment VI of liver cannot be discerned in current study, suggestive of regression.
The small cysts in segments IV and VIII show no interval change in appearance. There is no newly arised hepatic mass.
The portal veins are patent.
Pancreas, spleen and adrenal glands are normal.
The left renal artery is occluded with thrombi and the left kidney is small with absence of normal perfusion. This is a recent development since last CT scan. The right kidney is normal.
No ascites or intra-abdominal adenopathy is discerned.

OPINIONS:
The previously noted **intrahepatic** metastasis has regressed completely on imaging.
Thrombi in left renal **artery** causing chronic infarction and atrophy of left kidney.

ADVERSE REACTION:
Nil reported.

Reported by : DR. ▓▓▓   13/12/2007 11:41

Report to : ▓▓▓
Requested by : ▓▓▓   **Printed on** : 26/02/2008 10:08

Page 1 of 1

♪ 2007 年 12 月 13 日检查报告显示肝转移病灶等完全消失

牛奶产品的利弊

近30年来，营养学有突破性进展，对牛奶的研究已累积大量文献，关于牛奶致癌的研究指出：牛奶可能导致乳腺癌、卵巢癌、大肠癌等系列癌症。还有多项研究指出，牛奶及乳制品消费增加了男性前列腺癌发生的危险度。

2004年10月《新英格兰医学杂志》发表了一篇牛奶致女性乳腺癌的研究报道。丹麦的研究人员对117 000名妇女调查发现，牛奶对乳腺癌的促发有很大影响。研究人员认为，近50年来全世界乳腺癌发病率的大幅提高与人们饮食结构中牛奶及乳制品消费增加密切相关。大量饮用牛奶会增加人体中类胰岛素一号增长因数（IGF-Ⅰ）的水准，已经有多项研究表明，几乎每一种癌症都与IGF-Ⅰ有关联，IGF-Ⅰ是一种促使癌细胞生长和繁殖的关键性因素。

◇ 现代化生产牛奶激素过量

这其中有几个重要原则问题需要提出和思考。

(1) 现代化大规模饲养的奶牛与以往自然状态下生长的奶牛有很大不同。

(2) 现代化饲养的奶牛所生产的牛奶与自然状态下奶牛所生产的牛奶有很大的差异。

(3) 现代化生产的牛奶产品与自然状态下的奶牛所生产的牛奶，成分有很大的差异。

下面我们来看看这些差异和不同。

现代奶牛畜牧中，奶牛在生产后 3 个月即可进行人工授精，以人工授精替代了自然交配，使奶牛几乎在整个怀孕期间持续泌乳，尤其是妊娠后期，其血清中雌激素水平显著提高，牛奶中的雌激素也随之增加。据估计大约 75% 的商业化牛奶来源于妊娠奶牛。另一方面，为了提高产量，奶牛养殖者会给奶牛注射激素催奶剂，人工诱导奶牛泌乳。

◇ 高蛋白饲料

为增加牛奶产量，奶牛养殖者可能减少使用牧草饲养奶牛，而用含动物蛋白的高蛋白饲料饲养，这些高蛋白饲料改变了传统牛奶的含量成分，使激素的含量大大增加。

167

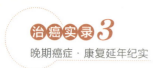

◇ 催乳剂

有些奶牛场给奶牛注射"控孕催乳剂"，使奶牛不怀孕就大量产奶，其产量竟然能够达到自然产奶量的10倍之多。他们还会给奶牛注射生长激素，使用了"奶牛激素"之后，可明显增高产量。为追求经济效益，一些奶牛饲养企业想尽办法改变千百年传统的奶牛养殖方法，导致奶牛激素过量。

2004年，瑞典卡洛林斯卡研究完成了一项牛奶与癌症的研究。研究证明，大量饮用牛奶导致妇女患卵巢癌。他们对61 084名年龄在38岁至76岁的妇女跟踪13年调查，确诊爱喝牛奶的266名妇女患卵巢癌，125名尚未确诊。每天饮用4次以上乳制品的妇女，卵巢癌的发病率比每天喝2次的妇女高出一倍。

美国国家癌症研究所的研究也发现牛奶内的雌激素、雄激素和胰岛素样生长因子（IGFs）就是主要致癌物质。加拿大的肿瘤专家建议，除了那些发展中国家的儿童和营养不良的成人，一般人并不需要喝太多牛奶。

◇ 牛奶制品导致性早熟

性早熟是大量饮用牛奶产品的另一副作用。

青春期前儿童体内产生雌激素少，对于外源性激素敏感性较高，暴露于外源性激素之中是非常危险的，可能使其生长加速或出现乳房发育等。一项国外的研究表明，对幼年雌鼠注射雌二醇会导致小鼠性早熟。

◇ 添加剂污染奶品

美国对肿瘤研究有贡献的医学教授新谷宏实经过四十多年的行医实践，以医疗实证为依据，充分证明牛奶会导致妇女乳腺癌。他在《不生病的生活》中告诉人们，他的法宝就是在患者做了肿瘤切除术之后，至少五年禁食牛奶和肉、鱼、蛋。他还指出"如果用市面上销售的牛奶代替母牛的乳汁来哺育小牛，那么小牛四五十天就有可能死掉"。科学家研究认为，加工奶经过均质化工艺和高温灭菌处理，乳脂和许多生物酶被破坏并变成了有害物质，这样的奶实际是一种"变质物"。牛吃了吸收不到营养并会慢性中毒，因此不久就会死亡。

以往农庄的鲜奶乳汁浓郁，没有掺水，走近农庄就能闻到飘逸的天然奶香。然而，当今的奶品市场是极少有这样的鲜奶的。大量的奶都是加工奶，而加工奶品确实有许多毒素。爱丁堡的约翰·汤姆森曾用孪生小牛做实验，一只喂鲜奶，另一只喂加工过的奶，吃鲜奶的小牛生长健康，吃加工奶的小牛在60天内死亡。实验重复了很多次，都得到了一样的结果。

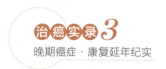

各种牛奶产品中的添加剂也很多，即使是儿童牛奶也少不了各式各样的添加剂。奶制品在包装上就有大量赫然明示的化学添加物质，例如香精、色素、阿斯巴甜、枸橼酸钠、黄原胶、三聚磷酸钠、纽红、苯丙氨酸、低聚糖、乳化剂、水分保持剂、增稠剂、酸度调节剂、日落黄等。这些添加剂也可能对身体产生不好的影响，如磷酸钠类添加剂，虽然可以让奶产品的口感更好，但会妨碍钙铁锌等微量元素的吸收。

◇ 奶制品不适宜乳腺癌等患者

在此，我们讲一个亲身经历的故事。

有位晚期乳腺癌患者全身大量器官（如双肺、脑、肝脏等）都有转移灶，主诊医生告知家人只有几周的生命，医院已经放弃治疗而前来就诊。在经过一年左右的生命修复治疗后，她的病情明显好转、稳定，长期低热早已退去，饮食恢复正常，日常生活正常，精神状态良好。但继之病情突然加重，我们完全不能找到原因。后来反复详细地追问这位患者和她的家属，例如在家中每天吃什么食物，做哪些工作等，才得知她不仅大量饮用牛奶，竟然还饮用骆驼奶，并且已经长达两个月了。非常震惊之余，我们产生了很多疑问，比如骆驼奶难道可以供给人饮用吗？香港不是沙漠地区，也不是牧区，香港人是怎样吃到骆驼奶的？骆驼产奶难道不喂给骆驼宝宝饮吗？那么骆驼宝宝会不会饿死？怎样捕获骆驼并且得到它的奶呢？

百思不得其解之后，试着在网上搜寻一下，才知道自己太落后了。原来骆驼奶不但有大量生产，而且早就打入市场了，是内地的朋友送给香港患者骆驼奶以便"增加营养"。骆驼也早就像奶牛一样饲养起来并进行着种种提高骆驼奶产量的激素注射了。因此现代化生产的牛奶制品是不能作为给癌症患者的营养品长期使用的，特别是乳腺癌、卵巢癌、前列腺癌等患者。

这些活生生的事实说明，人们为了经济利益越来越多地违背自然规律，自以为进步而实际在走向倒退。导致许多疾病发生发展的现代产业是需要社会去管理的，现代科技的发展和发达在一些方面是将人类引向愚昧无知、引向迫害自己，希望人人都担起一份责任来维护这个地球的生态。

恶性黑色素瘤多发淋巴转移，坚持抗癌 11 年

陈先生 47 岁时，偶感到左耳部和耳下方肿胀疼痛，以后越来越严重，导致进食困难，听力也受到了影响。他于 2007 年 6 月作左耳部肿瘤的切除，经病理学检查确诊为恶性黑色素瘤，并有腮腺、舌下腺等转移，当时医生说切除的面积比较大，希望不要复发，但是于 2008 年又发生淋巴结转移，陈先生急忙来

进行生命修复的中医药治疗。经过服用中药一段时间后，肿大的淋巴结消失，陈先生也就放心了。但是于2012年，又发现肺部有结节，双肺都有肿大的淋巴结，而且在气管前、纵隔等发现有肺部转移的可能性，陈先生急忙又来服用中药治疗。他当时咳嗽、多痰、胸闷、腹胀等，经生命修复治疗后，不适的症状逐渐消失，精神逐渐恢复正常。

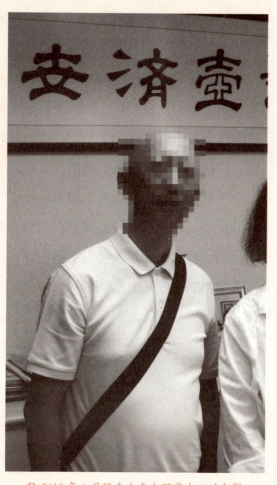

● 2018 年 6 月陈先生来本研究中心时合影

治疗原则

排毒化浊，祛瘀抗癌。

治疗方案

(1) 常用中药：土茯苓、生大黄、薏苡仁、猫爪草、藤梨根、牡丹皮、半枝莲、野菊花、丹参、虎杖等。

(2) 攻毒散同时服用。

时至现在，11 年已经过去了，陈先生坚持抗癌治疗，生活工作正常。

恶性黑色素瘤，在中医古代著作中被称为"黑子""脱疽""恶疮"等病，一般认为预后不良。

如《外科正宗》中记载："黑子，痣名也。此肾中浊气混滞于阳，阳气收束，结成黑子，坚而不散。凡人生此，终为不吉。"

恶性黑色素瘤为典型的通过血液发生转移的肿瘤，发展速度快，病情凶险，若治疗不及时，患者极易死亡。实际上，常规的治疗是很难达到遏制恶性黑色素瘤进展的疗效。我们运用中医排毒化浊、祛瘀抗癌的方法，使得患者可以长期正常生活，取得了明显的治疗效果。

附：患者相关检查报告

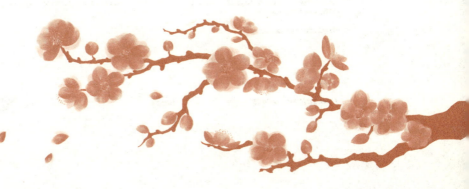

173

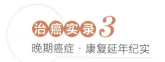

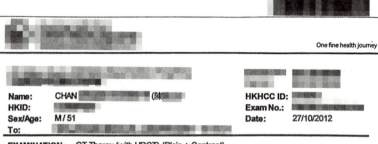

One fine health journey

Name:	CHAN ___ (陈___	**HKHCC ID:**	
HKID:		**Exam No.:**	
Sex/Age:	M / 51	**Date:**	27/10/2012
To:			

EXAMINATION: CT Thorax (with HRCT) (Plain + Contrast)

Report:

TECHNIQUES:

- Pre and post contrast scan of thorax performed.
- 100ml Iopamiro370 as IV contrast agent.
- Axial images of 5mm slice thickness in both mediastinum and lung window settings provided.
- HRCT axial images of 1mm slice thickness in lung window setting provided.

FINDINGS:

Mild fibrosis and pleural thickening in bilateral lung apices. Small non calcified lung nodules in left oblique fissure (2.6mm), left lingular segment (3.4mm) and right middle lobe (1.9mm). Features might represent post inflammatory granuloma. Follow up with cross sectional imaging to monitor the interval change in size of these lung nodules would be useful for further characterization.
The trachea and bronchi are patent.

Mediastinum and hilar shadow are wihtin normal limits. Small lymph nodes in pretracheal region (3.7mm), precarinal region (4.2mm) and prevascular space (7.1mm x 1.2cm), suggestive of reactive nodes.

The cardiac chambers are of normal size. Normal pulmonary vasculature noted. Major intrathoracic vessels are also patent.

There is no evidence of pleural thickening or effusion.

Liver covered in this examination shows hypodense lesion (1.9cm x 1.5cm) in segment VII/VI with suspicious mural enhancement. Correlation with ultrasound liver or CT or MRI upper abdomen with contrast would be useful for further characterization. Portal vein and hepatic vein are normally opacified.
No gallstone noted. Gallbladder wall not thickened. No evidence of pericholecystic fluid.
The spleen covered in the examination is normally enhanced, with no focal lesion seen. Adrenals are of normal density and contour with no focal lesion seen.
Kidneys covered in the examination show no focal lesion.
Small lymph nodes in portocaval region (up to 1.1cm) and aortocaval region (6.1mm), suggestive of reactive nodes.

No lytic bone lesion seen.

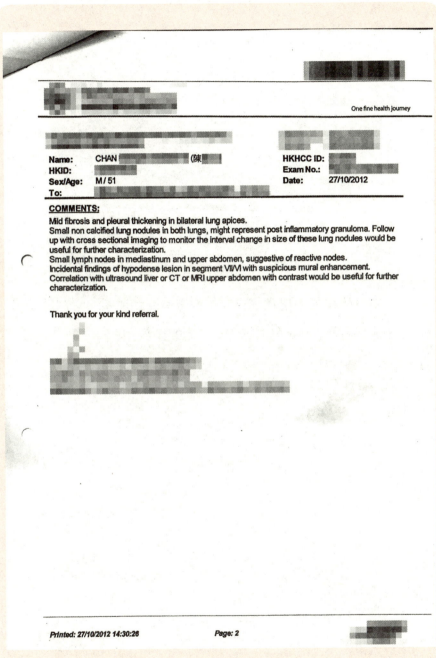

One fine health journey

Name: CHAN　　　　　(陳　　　　　　**HKHCC ID:**
HKID:
Sex/Age: M / 51　　　　　　　　　　**Exam No.:**
To:　　　　　　　　　　　　　　　　**Date:** 27/10/2012

COMMENTS:

Mild fibrosis and pleural thickening in bilateral lung apices.
Small non calcified lung nodules in both lungs, might represent post inflammatory granuloma. Follow up with cross sectional imaging to monitor the interval change in size of these lung nodules would be useful for further characterization.
Small lymph nodes in mediastinum and upper abdomen, suggestive of reactive nodes.
Incidental findings of hypodense lesion in segment VII/VI with suspicious mural enhancement.
Correlation with ultrasound liver or CT or MRI upper abdomen with contrast would be useful for further characterization.

Thank you for your kind referral.

Printed: 27/10/2012 14:30:26　　　　　　　*Page: 2*

🎧 2012 年 10 月 27 日检查报告显示双肺结节，胸膜增厚，纵隔及腹部淋巴结，肝部有结节病灶

175

解毒排毒

中医传统的治疗八法，都与排毒有密切关系。解毒排毒也是调整阴阳、平衡气血、化解疾病的重要方法。

◇ 汗法

借助出汗的方式来疏通人体经脉，加速血液循环，排出体内毒素。通过运动或者服用发散寒邪的中药通过发汗排出体内聚积的毒素代谢产物。

◇ 吐法

利用药食将毒物、痰涎等催吐出来。如果误食了药物或霉变、有毒食品，在胃中停留不久者，以吐法最简便。金元四大家之一的张子和就主张祛邪以安正，指出"凡上行者，皆吐法也。"

◇ 下法

对于毒邪积蓄的实症，或胃肠道里有腐败食物或毒素而体质不太虚者，可用下法，即用泻下法清除毒素。

◇ 和法

疾病在少阳半表半里，出现口苦、咽干、目眩等寒热及相

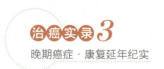
应症状，可用和解之法，以和解阴阳失调、消除病邪，使脏腑气血归于平衡。

◇ 温法

用温散寒邪的药物来进行治疗的方法，主要用于虚寒体征。寒证有表寒、里寒的不同，有寒在皮肤、经络、脏腑的不同，又有不同经络，不同脏腑的区别，温法的祛邪排毒用药也随之不同。

◇ 清法

清热解毒之法适用于清除热毒。患者出现发热、口干舌燥、咽喉肿痛、身体疼痛或不同经络、脏腑的火热、热毒之症，常用清法，即清理邪热毒邪之法。

◇ 消法

适用于消食除滞、化积消瘤等方面，是针对气、血、痰、食、水、虫等积聚的毒邪，使之消散的方法。凡食积、痞块、积聚、蓄水、痰核、瘰疬等皆可用消法。

◇ 补法

正气不足，就无力排毒祛邪，补法以补正为主，有补气、补血、补阴、补阳等，以扶助正气，祛除毒邪。

八法治疗是在辨证的基础上使用的，是历代经验的总结，是切合实际的治疗方法。

病案 17

晚期肺癌放弃化疗 15 年

潘先生是位成功的企业家，他在香港有制衣公司，制造名牌男女服装，远销欧洲各国，近几年来他又向国内投资，发展酒店、旅游业等。潘先生是大老板，他手下有各个部门的经理、职工人员众多，大家都认为老板工作认真、精明、精力充沛，对员工要求严格，一点小毛病也会被他发现，更不敢有过失，否则就会担心被炒鱿鱼。但是对潘老

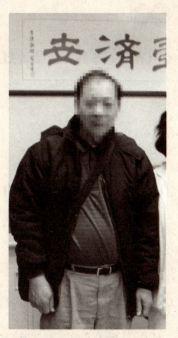

🎧 2018 年 4 月潘先生来研究中心留念

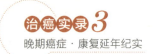
板，新来的年轻人不知道而只有老员工才知道的事情是，原来这位老板患肺癌并发展到晚期，至今已有 15 年多了。

潘先生于 2002 年年底发现肺癌，那时他 62 岁，发现后立即在正规的大医院进行当时最先进的靶向治疗。但是用西药 3 个月后，肺部肿瘤没有缩小，而且还转移到了胸膜上，病情加重，肺部和胸膜都有癌肿，已属晚期。潘先生果断放弃西医治疗，前来进行生命修复的中医药治疗。当时他胸痛严重，呼吸短促，咳嗽频繁，自己和家人都感到病情严重不容乐观。

益气养阴，排毒，散结消瘤。

治疗方案

(1) 常用中药：瓜蒌、薤白、太子参、黄药子、生地黄、玉竹、石斛、玄参、川贝、浙贝母、生大黄、全蝎等。

(2) 散结丸同时服用。

经辨证分析，我们采用了益气、排毒攻癌、软坚散结为治的中医药治疗，几个月后，他的病情明显好转，疼痛基本消失，其他症状也明显改善。他因工作繁忙，没有耐心，对此病也缺乏充分的认识，遂停止治疗，不再吃中药。但一个月后病情再次加重，咳嗽并出现咯血、胸痛背痛，于是急忙又前来治疗，不敢再停药。

这样又坚持一年左右后，经检查双肺肿瘤消失，没有出现新的转移病灶，潘先生仍坚持治疗数年，此后改为间断服药，至今他仍努力工作，肿瘤也没有复发。

肺癌是发病率死亡率很高的癌症，晚期肺癌更是凶险，肺癌也是我们治疗最多的癌症之一。这些成功治疗的案例说明，癌症和晚期癌症都是可治的。不仅仅是化疗、靶向治疗、放射治疗等方法可用于治癌，更有中医药这样天然的无不良反应的、更有效的治疗方法可供选择。

附：患者相关检查报告

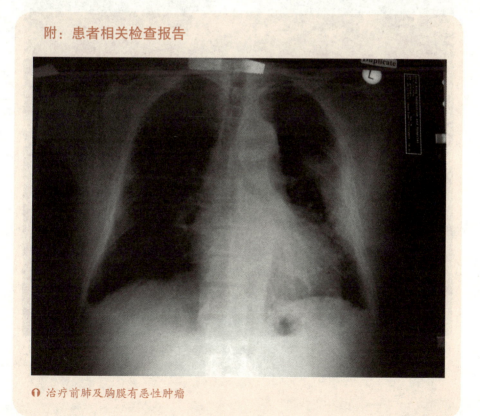

↑ 治疗前肺及胸膜有恶性肿瘤

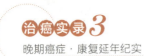

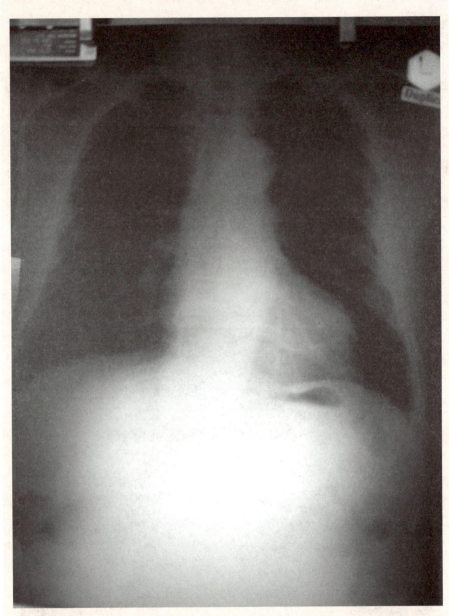

❶ 治疗后肺部肿瘤已消失

Hospital
Scanning Department
(CT, MR, NM, PET Scan, Bone Densitometry)

Tel: ▮▮▮▮▮▮▮▮▮▮▮▮ Fax: ▮▮▮▮▮▮

REPORT FOR MRI/CT/NM/PET SCANNING EXAMINATION

OUR REF. : ▮▮▮▮▮▮▮▮▮▮

NAME : Pun ▮▮▮▮▮

ID No. : E2▮▮▮▮▮

EXAM. DATE : Wed, 23 Feb, 2005

There is no abnormal hypermetabolic lesion in the head and neck and supraclavicular fossae. Bilateral axillae are normal.

The liver shows uniform physiological activity. Bilateral adrenals are normal. No significant positive finding is present in the abdomen and pelvis.

There is no focal lesion in the axial bony skeleton.

(The plain CT images are performed for anatomical correlation and localization of lesion seen on PET. This is not a complete diagnostic contrast CT study).

IMPRESSION :

Good clinical response when compared with the pretreatment study in 17 June 2004. No residual active tumor nodule is present in both lungs. No residual hypermetabolic lymph node is present in the thorax. No evidence of metastasis is noted in the brain, head and neck, thorax, abdomen and pelvis.

SIGNED:

DR REPORT

⋂ 2005 年 2 月 23 日 PET−CT 检查报告与 2004 年 6 月 17 日检查比较，对治疗反应良好，两肺未见有肿瘤，胸部无肿大淋巴结，脑、颈、胸、骨盆均无转移病灶

排毒途径

◇ 将毒素排出体外

在人类历史的漫长岁月中，人是在没有大量化学污染的环境中逐步发展的，所以在不断进化的过程中，人身体的排毒系统主要用来清除体内代谢过程中所产生的毒素，而用它清除外来的人工毒素、化学物质等并不有效，至少至今还没有发展出这方面的特别功能。如通过工业排放或吸烟，导致重金属或毒素进入身体，它们就将长期存在于体内，可能诱发肺癌等癌症疾病。

进入身体中的毒素，一部分长期滞留在体内有关组织中，一部分可以通过粪便、尿液、汗液和呼吸通道直接排出，一部分可以通过肝脏先解毒再行排出，但仍有许多毒素需要通过治疗的方法来强化人体的排毒功能，从而更有效的排出毒素。

排毒就是排出体内毒素或避免毒素进入体内。我们需要避免来自食物、药物和环境方面的毒素，并及时排出体内代谢废物等毒素。食物中的毒素包括残留的化肥、农药、激素、兽药、添加剂、反式脂肪及转基因成分等。药物中的毒素来自常用止痛药、抗生素、类固醇及各种对症药物如减肥药、降糖药、降压药和抗肿瘤药物等。环境中的毒素来自空气污染、水污染、建筑装修材料、印刷品、洗涤剂、化妆品和其他日化用品等。

人体的循环系统由心血管系统和淋巴系统组成。心血管系统主要负责运送血液和营养物质，而淋巴系统则主要负责运送不被利用的废物，因此被称为身体的下水道。

毒素在体内累积过多，除了会导致疾病之外，也会影响人体的气血运行、代谢平衡、脏腑功能、精神状态、皮肤气色，并会加速

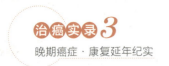

人体老化。因此，有效抵御外毒并排出内毒是维护健康的重要内容。

1. 饮水排毒

饮用天然矿泉水或过滤纯净水。每天饮用足够量的水，养成定时饮水的习惯。水可以提高酶的活性和分子化学反应速度，改善代谢和循环，稀释毒素并有助于毒素排出。

2. 毛孔排毒

排出毒素的其中一个通道是汗腺，而桑拿、温泉浴、药浴等是促进汗腺排毒最有效的方法。因为它不仅可以提升体温，提高酶的数量和活性，促进血液和淋巴循环，增加氧气供应，而且能够打开汗腺，带出体内毒素。汗水可以稀释带走部分水溶性的毒素，也包括一些重金属、油脂等脂溶性的毒素。

3. 皮肤排毒

外界的毒素许多是接触皮肤的，体内的一些毒素又是通过皮肤排出的，所以清洗是直接的皮肤排毒法。

4. 胃肠道排毒

通过洗胃、灌肠、洗肠、服用中药等方法可以排出消化道积蓄的毒素。

5. 螯合排毒

运用螯合技术选取有一定功能的物质，使之在体内与重金属等不同毒素结合，然后排出体外。

6. 运动排毒

运动使得血液循环加速，通过心跳加快、呼吸加速、毛孔开放、新陈代谢增加等方法，借呼吸、皮肤、大小便等多种途径，促进体内多种毒素排出。

晚期乳腺癌多发转移，与癌抗争 19 年

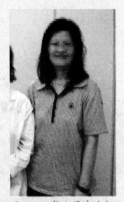

🔊 2018 年 4 月丰小姐
来研究中心合影留念

丰小姐是一家公司的文员，每日循规蹈矩地从家里到办公室上班，再从办公室下班回家。她原以为这种生活很平淡正常，并无很大的奢望。但是工作中也常有不顺心如意之处，个人生活比较单调，40 多岁了，还是独身一人。她于 1999 年常感到右侧乳房部位及上肢牵拉绷紧不适，去医院检查，以为打针吃药就好了，没想到竟然查出患了乳腺癌。于是她于 1999 年 5 月做了右侧乳腺肿瘤切除手术，手术后又继续进行了几年的内分泌治疗，虽然有许多副作用，她还是坚持下来了。以后以为没事了，却又发现了左乳腺癌，又于 2008 年初做了左乳腺切除。接着又做了化疗、放疗。

尽管如此，她说该做的都做了，但是于 2009 年初又发现了双肺的阴影以及乳腺手术部位皮肤转移、溃破结节。常规的治疗方法已经都做完了，医院讲生命也不会很久了。她只好前来寻求生命修复的治疗。

当时她气促、胸闷、咳嗽频繁、气短难续。当时的治疗原则是解毒散结，破滞消瘤。

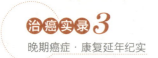

解毒散结，破滞消瘤。

治疗方案

(1) 常用中药：三棱、莪术、藤梨根、生大黄、枳实、厚朴、山慈菇、黄药子、浙贝母、败酱草等。

(2) 散结丸同时服用。

随着治疗时间的推移，她逐渐症状减轻，没有气短咳嗽，并在长达一年的时间内坚持治疗，与癌抗争，此后慢慢恢复了健康。到如今，已一切正常，她在抗癌路上已顺利地走过了 19 年。

乳腺癌并不是现代病，在中医古籍中称为"乳岩"，因为肿块坚硬如岩石，凹凸不平而得名。古代医书已对乳腺癌有详细的描述。明代医书《外科正宗》中记载："忧郁伤肝，思虑伤脾，积想在心，所愿不得志者，致经络痞涩，聚结成核，初如豆大，始生痛疼，渐若棋子。半年一年，二载三载，不疼不痒，渐渐而大，始生疼痛，痛则无解，日后肿如堆栗，或如复碗，紫色气秽，渐渐溃烂，深者如岩穴，凸者若泛莲，疼痛连心，出血则臭，其时五脏俱衰，四大不救，名曰乳岩"。生命修复治疗晚期乳腺癌的原则与治疗其他晚期癌症一致，既治疗局部的肿瘤和转移病灶，更治疗整体。以改变癌症患者全身阴阳代谢整体失衡和改变体内适合癌细胞发展转移的癌环境为主要治疗手段，燮理阴阳，平调脏腑，攻毒抗癌。

附：患者相关检查报告

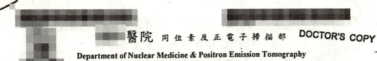

醫院 同位素及正電子掃描部 **DOCTOR'S COPY**

Department of Nuclear Medicine & Positron Emission Tomography

HOSPITAL

Name:	Fung, ▉ 馮▉		Date:	12/08/2009
I.D. No.:	▉	Sex: Female	Ref. Dr.:	
Hosp. No.:		Age: 51 Y	Fax:	▉
Ward/Dept.:			Tel:	

POSITRON EMISSION TOMOGRAPHY
(^{18}F-FDG ONCOLOGY)

History:

A 51 year-old lady had MRM for pTisN0 carcinoma of right breast in 05/1999 followed by Tamoxifen till 06/2002. She developed left breast malignancy, T1bN2 disease, treated with BCT in 03/2008. Patient was given adjuvant chemoradiation therapy completed by 02/2009, followed by Femara. Recent chest x-ray showed opacity in left and right mid zone with air bronchogram. She complained of exertional dyspnea and cough. History of crack fractured right forearm in 04/2009 and excision of chocolate cyst. Non-diabetic. No TB.

Radiopharmaceutical: 12.6 mCi F-18 Fluorodeoxyglucose (^{18}FDG) injected intravenously.

Findings:

Limited whole body CT transmission and PET emission imaging began at 70 minutes after radiopharmaceutical administration (blood glucose 5.6 mmol/l), spanning a region from base of skull to upper thigh. 60 mg Spasmonal was given p.o. 15 min before ^{18}FDG administration.

Liver tissue normal reference uptake has a SUVmax of 3.64 and delayed SUVmax of 3.34.

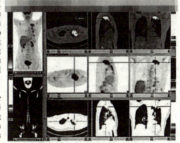

Patient is status post right MRM and left BCT. Mild patchy ^{18}FDG activity with delay decrease metabolism is seen along the subcutaneous region of left breast, suggestive of inflammation. No discrete focal metabolic activity in remaining left breast or right chest wall to suggest local recurrent disease. No hypermetabolic lymphadenopathies are demonstrated in bilateral axillae, internal mammary chains or supraclavicular fossae.

Partial consolidations, patchy lung density and air bronchogram with moderate increased ^{18}FDG activities are seen in left anterior lung field, worst in the apical region, suggestive of pneumonitic changes. A mildly active left hilar node is present. No suspicious focal metabolism is seen in the right lung or remaining mediastinum.

There is no abnormal focal glycolysis in nasopharynx, thyroid and upper cervical nodes. Liver shows uniform uptake without focal area of hypermetabolism. Spleen, adrenal glands and pancreas appear unremarkable. There is mild focal ^{18}FDG activity over the splenic flexure of colon. No hypermetabolic lymphadenopathy is demonstrated in the abdomen or pelvis. There is no suspicious focal metabolic activity in the uterine area. Skeletal survey shows no abnormal focal uptake to suggest active osseous metastasis.

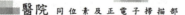

醫院 同位素及正電子掃描部

Department of Nuclear Medicine & Positron Emission Tomography

HOSPITAL

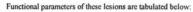

Functional parameters of these lesions are tabulated below:

Fung,		in mm		Standard	Delayed
Site		LD	PD	SUVmax	SUVmax
Lt apex		54.2	44.6	11.0	13.6
Lt anteromedial lung field		38.8	12.5	4.9	6.0
Lt hilar		12.3	7.7	3.4	3.4
Mild patchy uptake in Lt breast		12.5	10.3	2.3	1.8
Splenic flexure		14.1	9.4	5.1	-

Note: LD=longest diameter; PD=diameter perpendicular to LD

Impression:

1. Partial consolidations with patchy lung density and increased ^{18}FDG activity in left anterior lung field, worst on the apical aspect. The overall scintigraphic pictures are suggestive of post-irradiation pneumonitis. Metastatic focus is less favor though cannot be entirely excluded. Follow-up scan is recommended.
2. The mildly active left hilar node should carry similar pathology as in left anterior lung field.
3. Non-specific inflammation over the subcutaneous region of left breast. Otherwise, no metabolic evidence of local recurrent disease in left breast or right chest wall. No regional metastatic lymphadenopathy.
4. Incidental findings of mild focal activity over the splenic flexure of colon. Findings can be explained by focal inflammation or early dysplastic polyp. Colonoscopy or follow up scan for progress may be helpful for differentiation, or as clinically indicated.

Thank you very much, _____ for your referral.

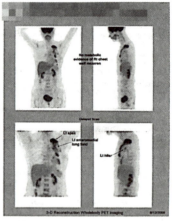

🎧 2009年8月12日检查报告示双乳癌，肺部阴影等病灶，并有肺门淋巴结、皮下、结肠部病灶等

快乐抗癌

　　人类抗击肿瘤历史悠久。近 100 年来，手术、化疗、放疗等治疗手段相继问世，免疫治疗、靶向治疗、基因治疗等治疗新技术亦层出不穷。在一系列对肿瘤的攻克过程中，还应该重视精神因素及情绪与癌症的关系。

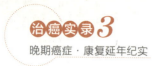

◇ "癌症性格"

癌症性格是指一些特定的、不良的性格特点如神经质、易怒、悲观或是孤僻的人更容易成为癌魔狩猎的对象，而开朗乐观则有助于预防和治疗癌症。

有不少调查发现，癌症好发于一些受到挫折后，长期处于精神压抑、焦虑、沮丧、苦闷、恐惧、悲哀、紧张等情绪的人。

中医学认为"七情"过度会导致气血运行障碍而生病，认为"百病皆生于气""万病皆源于心"。

有研究表明，精神心理因素并不能直接致癌，但它却往往以一种慢性的持续性的刺激来影响和降低机体的免疫力，提高癌症的发生率。与此相反，乐观的精神、良好的情绪、积极的心理状态能增强大脑皮质和神经系统的功能，使免疫系统发挥正常作用。也有研究指出，癌症患者的免疫系统存在一定的缺陷，因此，良好的心态对于免疫系统发挥正常功能有良好的作用。

◇ 不良情绪可诱发肿瘤并加速肿瘤生长

常见于癌症患者的典型精神情绪特征如下。

(1) 长期背负精神压力，无法缓解。精神压力来自于工作、生活、人际关系等各方面。患者往往对压力承受能力差，常常不能恰当应对这类压力，一般不轻易说出，往往隐藏着这种精神压力。

(2) 严重的心理创伤使精神受到打击，使人脆弱或消沉，性格发生改变。

(3) 长时间悲伤的情绪，如对于亲人的去世、经济的损失、上当受骗的打击等经常想起，念念不忘。

(4) 过度的嫉妒心态，总觉得不如自己的人得到了更好的待遇，世界对于自己太不公道。

(5) 其他长期不良情绪。如长期抑郁、心情沮丧、过度思虑而不能缓解，易导致的失眠、食欲差、精神障碍等问题。

有项调查发现，80%以上的癌症患者在患病前曾遭受过负面生活事件的打击，如配偶死亡、夫妻不和、生活规律重大改变、工作学习压力大、子女管教困难、夫妻两地分居等。北京、上海等大城市的一项398例胃癌配对调查发现，各地患者都有一个共同点，即胃癌患者都有经常生闷气的情况。

国外也有学者发现，癌症是一种与精神心理因素有着密切关系的疾病。长期爱较真、拘谨、不轻易表达自己的情感、经常压抑愤怒不满等情绪的人更容易患胃癌。而在女性脑瘤与淋巴瘤患者中，大多都有内向、孤僻的性格特点。总是追求尽善尽美甚至吹毛求疵的人其心率通常比别人快，且容易睡不好或失眠，消化系统功能较弱，比常人更容易得消化道癌及肺癌。在乳腺癌患者中，也有不少是"完美主义者"，对人对己的要求都特别高，如过分追求完美，凡事爱较真，常常钻牛角尖，过分在意别人的评论眼光，过度压抑自己的情绪，不善发泄和表达，生活工作争强好胜，使内分泌系统长期处在高度亢奋状态等。

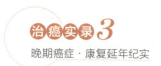

德国的科学家巴尔特鲁斯博士曾经对 8000 例癌症患者进行调查，发现患者得癌前 1 ～ 2 年大多都出现过忧郁、焦虑、失望和难以解脱的情绪变化，大多数患者在涉及失望、孤独及其他沉重打击和精神压力频繁发生之后发病。

◇ 压力与创伤的宣泄和释放

虽然很多人都会经历压力、创伤、冲突、悲伤及失败等事件，大多数人可以认识到这些不愉快的经历甚至打击都是生活中的常见挑战，经过缓冲，会逐渐缓解、淡忘、平静下来。而对于有些人来说，则很容易受到这些压力和创伤的伤害，无法从悲伤、痛苦、愤怒或忿恨的困扰中解脱出来，无法缓解压力，甚至会绵延持久提升压力水平。

相当一些患者当遭遇这些创伤时，容易陷入创伤及痛苦的感情经历不能自拔。压力激素皮质醇水平迅速上升，保持在高水平，这会直接抑制免疫系统，造成体内癌症生长恶化。

因此，我们要学会合理宣泄心中的不快，学会倾诉，学会向身边的人表达自己的情感，千万别做"闷葫芦"，内心的压力长时间得不到释放，就会削弱身体的免疫功能，给癌症以可乘之机。

如何释放压力？患者应该换一种思维方式，完美与不完美往往只在一念之间。要想活得健康些，有时不妨过得稍稍糊涂些。与其事事都看得太重，不如学着分清主次，有张有弛。重要的事情及时做、认真做；较重要的事情努力做；不重要的事情不必急着做。

应当了解释放压力的方法，如向朋友、家人倾诉，转移培养自己的新的兴趣爱好，运动、养花、弹琴、听音乐……总之让心情放松下来就能有效地释放压力。

◇ **勇敢面对癌症的挑战**

一般说来，恶性肿瘤患者的心理演变有规律可循。

没有确诊之前，恐惧和急于证实的心理占主导。焦虑、不安情绪为基本表现。发现不好的"苗头"，奔走于多家医院之间。检查确诊，特别希望虚惊一场，但心怀巨大恐惧。心理相当矛盾，睡不好、吃不好、精神不好，这些都有可能使病情加重。

一旦确诊，初期表现为恐惧、回避、否定的心理特征。患者当知道自己得的是癌症后，恐惧不安。当心态平静后便开始怀疑诊断正确与否，坐卧不安，要求多次检查确认。当患者明确自己患的是癌症时会变得愤怒沮丧、悲观绝望，甚至精神崩溃，病情急剧恶化。相当的患者也会随着时间推移，情绪开始慢慢平静，但有些却仍长期表现抑郁和悲伤。

任何一个人一旦被确诊为癌症，心理都将承受巨大压力，会发生一系列的心理反应。我们应尽量疏导这些心理反应，使患者平静而勇敢地面对现实以助于治疗。

研究也发现，一些战胜癌症的抗癌"明星"始终保持着乐

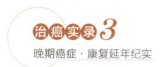
观自信的心态，这有助于治疗的效果，也说明了心理与免疫具有明显的相关性。

直系亲属是癌症患者最基本的社会支持来源，我们应该给患者创造一个有利康复的环境。家庭成员的状态对帮助患者实现每一步的治疗目标都非常重要，家属要积极参与患者的治疗过程，鼓励患者，对患者的需求做出及时、积极的反应，这样有利于患者积极面对疾病。已经战胜癌症，或者长期稳定、生活正常的患者给予新患者的鼓励和交流也很重要，大量的抗癌实例对患者树立信心很有帮助，这也是我们这系列抗癌书籍出版的主要目的。

◇ 快乐小鼠的研究

2010 年《细胞》杂志刊登了一个外国实验室的发现。给两组小鼠做相同的肿瘤种植实验，然后把一组小鼠放在一个"富足的生存环境"中，即在饲养笼子里放上各种小鼠喜爱的玩具，例如迷宫、玩具、滑轮、房子等，每个笼子中的小鼠数多于 8 只，保证它们尽情地互动。生活在这种状态下的小鼠被称为"快乐小鼠"。在红外线拍摄下，记者看到，小鼠不仅白天玩，在夜间也玩耍频繁，表现活跃；而对照组小鼠则显得平静甚至有些呆滞。

比较两组小鼠发现，"快乐小鼠"的肿瘤重量比对照组的都要低，有的肿瘤不仅变小，还消失了。实验涉及的黑色素瘤、胰腺癌、肺癌都有类似情况。其中，黑色素瘤抑瘤率 43.1%，

Pan02 胰腺癌的抑瘤率为 58.2%，Lewis 肺癌的抑瘤率为 36.5%。研究人员也在"快乐小鼠"的下丘脑发现了"脑来源神经营养因子"高表达。这项实验提示了良性精神刺激可能改变了癌细胞的代谢，同时影响到免疫系统。这也提示了精神行为对肿瘤的影响。

◇ 七情致病

中医学对七情致病有深刻的认识，其理论体系注重人的思想、情感、行为等心理因素与躯体疾病的相互关系，从一个重要方面揭示了疾病、癌症的病机。

《黄帝内经》中指出："百病生于气也，喜则气缓、怒则气上、忧则气聚、思则气结、悲则气消、恐则气下、惊则气乱。"可见七情所伤最容易致气机功能紊乱，从而形成气滞、气逆、气陷、气闭、气脱的病理状态，致使脏腑功能障碍，导致疾病的发生。

《金匮要略》指出，人有七情，即喜、怒、忧、思、悲、恐、惊。这些是生命中经常出现的情绪表现，但如果太过就会成为致病因素。

《素问·阴阳应象大论》说"怒伤肝""喜伤心""思伤脾""忧伤肺""恐伤肾"。《儒门集验方》云"盖五积者，因怒忧思七情之气，以伤五腑而成病也"。《灵枢五变》指出："内伤于忧怒而积聚成矣"。

由此看出：情绪的异常或过激会导致气血状态的改变。

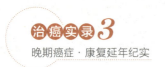

◇ 情绪变化导致气血运行失常

怒则气上，在发怒的时候，气血被导引向上，这时会出现怒发冲冠、怒目圆睁、声调高亢；思则气结，如果思虑过度、多疑、猜想、嫉妒等，则气血运行涩滞，脏腑功能失常，造成气滞血瘀，血脉凝泣。《灵枢·百病始生篇》说："气上逆则六俞不通，温气不行，凝血蕴里而不散……而积皆成矣。"

◇ 情绪波动造成气血病理改变

过度的不良情绪在发生的当时可使气血逆乱，反复发生之后，则会导致病理性改变且难以恢复。如果没有从心理上完全消除事件的影响，这种气血逆乱的病理改变会进一步造成脏腑功能失调。

情绪经常波动，不正常的气血逆乱会累积叠加。长期非生理状态的气血运行逆乱是导致病变的基础。

长期异常的情绪、行为变化导致气血亏虚，正气不足，因而难以抵抗外来病邪侵袭且可能内生疾病。

《内经》说："正气存内，邪不可干"，"邪之所凑，其气必虚"。疾病的发生与否除了与邪气的多少有关，还取决于正气的强弱。如果人的身体健康，免疫系统正常，是有对抗致病因素包括癌症的能力的。在七情中，悲伤和忧思耗伤正气；思虑过度伤脾，以致气机逆乱，精血不足，正气衰败。可见，不良的思想、情感、行为可降低人体免疫系统杀伤癌细胞的能力，导致癌症的发生。

从情志对五脏的影响来看，不同的情绪状态也可能导致特定脏器的癌变。例如对未来总是忧心忡忡，面对逆境过于消极悲观易患肺癌；遇事想不开、思虑过度，妒忌心强易患消化系统癌症等。

◇ 重视调理七情的治疗

中医学强调整体观、以阴阳五行理论作为指导，以人为本，调治内伤七情，调动患者内在的抗病积极因素，以达到促使患者康复，控制癌症转移的效果，这对预防癌症发生、发展、复发是很重要的。

癌症的发生发展多是情志不遂，气机不畅，久则影响五脏六腑的功能，使正气亏损，易致外邪入侵。气为血帅，气行则血行，气滞则血滞，致终成积聚。气血的正常运行，以及气血的正常生理状态，是生命的根本。气机阻滞、气滞血瘀、经络淤堵都与癌症的发生有密切相关，而情志失调是导致气血失调的重要原因之一。

情志太过和不及均可导致疾病，故而对情志的调治也可以治疗疾病。历代医家一直提倡"善医者，必先医其心，而后医其身。"突出了情志调治的首要性。他们从形神密不可分的观点出发，认为治疗疾病不仅要治其身，更要治其心。华佗说："夫

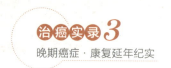
形者神之舍也，而精者气之宅也。舍坏则神荡，宅动则气散。神荡则昏，气散则疲。昏疲之身心，即疾病之媒介，是以善医者先医其心，而后医其身，其次则医其未病。"这里强调形神密不可分，并明确提出了身心健康的概念，比西方医学的身心健康概念要早 1700 年。

中医古籍早有"以情胜情"治病的记载，应用情志之间阴阳五行属性的对立互制调治七情。如孙思邈曰："世人欲识卫生道，喜乐有常，真怒少。"即教人常以喜乐胜悲怒，调治情志不遂，从而避免气机紊乱，维持脏腑气血的正常运行。对患者以理开导，减轻焦虑、苦闷、紧张等过激心理，解除患者心理负担，然后告之疾病之所害，讲明具体调治措施与方法，唤起患者的勇气与信心使其能够积极配合治疗，即《内经》所云："告之以其败，语之以其善，导之以其所便，开之以其所苦"。《续名医类案》云："失志不遂之病，非排遣性情不可"，"虑投其所好以移之，则病自愈"即指调节情志治疗可据患者个性、特长、文化修养的不同，鼓励患者转换环境接近自然，以排遣忧思、易转心志、养心悦身，从而促进康复。

◇ **注意情志调理**

1. 医生及家人都应该设法使患者心情舒畅

清代赵濂在《医门补要·人忽反常》中说："凡七情之喜惧爱憎，怡乎居室衣服，饮食好玩，皆与平昔迥乎相反者，殆非祸兆，即是病机，他人只可迎其意而宛然劝解，勿可再拂其性而使更剧也。"所以，应尽量创造条件，达到客观许可，尊重、体谅、同情、迁就患者情绪，适当满足患者愿望有助于癌症的治疗。

2. 利用五行生克的原理调理情志

分析五脏六腑的盛衰强弱，并按五行配五脏五志，利用情志之间的制约关系进行治疗。《素问·阴阳应象大论》中就提到可以用悲伤治疗愤怒，欣喜治疗悲伤，恐惧治疗狂喜，思考治疗恐惧，愤怒治疗思虑过度。《儒林外史》中范进中举的故事就是恐惧治疗狂喜的最好例证。癌症患者常常思虑过度，因此，可以让他们发泄心中的愤怒，以使各种情绪得以平衡协调。

3. 注意调摄精神和情绪锻炼

正如《素问·上古天真论》说："上古之人，其知道者，法于阴阳，和于术数，食饮有节，起居有常，不妄作劳"，"恬淡虚无，真气从之，精神内守，病安从来？"当人们面对纷繁复杂的世事时，能做到真诚、坦荡、宽容，即可使真气从之，精神内守，百病不能侵犯。

病案19

晚期胃癌加肠癌，健康生活 12 年

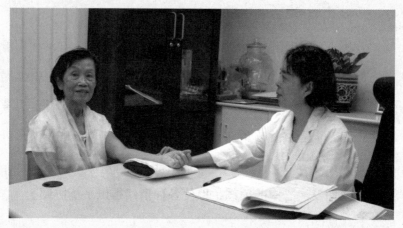

🎧 赵太太于 2018 年 6 月来研究中心留影

　　赵太太 80 岁了，2006 年因长期胃痛和呕吐到医院去做胃镜检查，经取组织活检，确诊为胃癌。又做了 CT 影像学检查，报告指出，除了已证实为胃癌外，肝脏有多发的结节，肺上也有 2 个结节，考虑有肝和肺转移。赵太太于 2006 年做了胃的部分切除手术，进行了化疗和放疗，因为医生和检查报告都指出有肝转移等。化疗放射治疗的过程非常痛苦，但她努力坚持下来。没想到即便做了这些痛苦的治疗，仍好景不长，于术后三年因腹痛去医院检查，又发现了肠癌并有多发的淋巴转移等。经检查，这是肠新发生的肿瘤，而不是转移而来，与以前的化疗、放疗等有关，需要再次手术。

赵太太很想知道她为什么这样不幸，为什么会患上两种癌症。经过多方了解和查阅书籍，终于明白化疗和放射治疗本身都有化学和放射毒害，本身就有导致癌症发生的可能。她在胃癌术后较长时间使用化疗和放射治疗，很有可能导致了第二种癌症的发生。赵太太又按照医生的要求，决定尽快再次做手术切除肠癌，就在即将做手术之前又有麻烦发生。她因为感染出现了急性肾衰竭，需要先洗肾才能够做手术。

首次手术以后，赵太太的体重减了10磅；第二次手术后，再减轻了10磅，这使她虚弱不堪，与之前判若两人，亲朋好友见到她都不敢相认。她自己也感到生命快到尽头。术后肾功能继续转差，癌指数却不断上升，肾功能更出现衰竭，无法再接受化疗和放射治疗。

在没有其他办法的情况下，赵太太前来求助于生命修复的抗癌中医药治疗。初诊时她的身体极度虚弱，由于呕吐、胀满，连中药也无法吞咽，只有安排抗癌及固本同时进行，少量多次地煎煮服用中药。来诊时见胸闷腹胀、嗳气频作、脘腹胀痛、时时呕吐、大便不畅、小便很少。

 治疗原则

通腑泄毒，通滞消瘤。

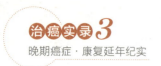

治疗方案

(1) 常用中药：人参、白术、山药、厚朴、大黄、芦荟、鸡内金、土鳖虫、地榆、重楼、土茯苓、虎杖、槐角等。

(2) 化癥丸同时服用。

六腑以通为用，患者胃腑肠道都出现恶性肿瘤，应行气化痰、通下。大黄、芦荟、厚朴、槟榔、地榆均为通腑泄毒的常用药，患者年老体弱，要同时顾及中气，故用人参、白术、山药等补药。鸡内金、土鳖虫、槟榔、香附等则用于行气通滞止痛、化瘀消瘤。

除了患有胃癌、肠癌及发生转移外，赵太太还有高血压、肾衰竭、腹痛、失眠、咳嗽、头晕、疲乏无力等症，全部要靠抗癌中医药治疗。当时医院就曾告诉她，因为她不能化疗，所以很快就会加重肺和肝的转移，生命非常危险。

计算一下，从患癌症至今已12年过去了。她坚持服用中药，身体良好，已没有任何不适。每次来看病时，问她有什么不舒服，她总是回答："什么都没有，能吃能睡，生活完全正常。"自从采用抗癌中医药治疗后，赵太太血压正常，肾功能正常，也没有发生医院里早就预言过的全身多脏器癌症转移及复发的情况。她有时也去医院进行常规检查，各项检查指标均为正常。她现在每日清晨都会像年轻人一样游泳锻炼，身体健康，心情愉快。

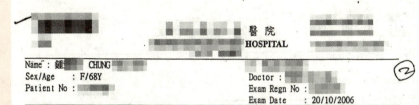

附：患者相关检查报告

醫 院
HOSPITAL

Name : 鍾　CHUNG

Sex/Age : F/68Y

Patient No :

Doctor :

Exam Regn No :

Exam Date : 20/10/2006

Exam : WHOLE ABDOMEN (P + C)

REPORT :

There is an ulcer crater with enhancing mucosal thickening demonstrated in the gastric pylorus which likely represents the biopsy proven malignant gastric ulcer. It measures about 1.56cm x 2.45cm x 4.93cm in size. There is associated nonspecific gastric wall thickening extending into the distal pyloric antrum. No gross extra-luminal tumour infiltration of the perigastric fat or adjacent structure demonstrated. No significant regional enlarged lymphadenopathy demonstrated.

There are two nonspecific small nodules in the left lung base (0.42cm and 0.25cm). No discrete focal lesion identified in the right lung base. No pleural effusion demonstrated.

No gross erosive bone lesion demonstrated. Small sclerotic foci in the pelvic girdle may represent small bone islands.

There are multiple well-defined hypodense hypoenhancing foci in both lobes of liver which may represent hepatic cysts, although cystic metastases from adenocarcinoma cannot be definitely excluded, the largest in the left lobe measures 1.66cm x 2.07cm x 1.54cm and the largest in the right lobe measures 1.08cm x 1.72cm x 1.63cm. No gross biliary ductal dilatation demonstrated. The portal veins, hepatic veins and IVC are patent. The gallbladder appears normal, no hyperdense gallstone demonstrated.

The pancreas is normal in size and configuration with normal homogeneous enhancement. The pancreatic duct is not dilated. The spleen is not enlarged. No gross adrenal mass lesion demonstrated.

Both kidneys are normal in size, position and axis of alignment. Smooth renal contour with no evidence of renal scarring. Preserved renal cortical thickness on both sides. No hyperdense urolithiasis or

C
T
S
C
A
N

Date: 20/10/2006 16:56

Page: 1 of 3　/cy

C.T. SCAN

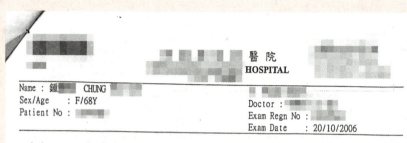

Name : 鍾███ CHUNG ███
Sex/Age : F/68Y
Patient No : ███

Doctor : ███
Exam Regn No : ███
Exam Date : 20/10/2006

hydroureteronephrosis demonstrated. Both kidneys show normal enhancement and contrast excretion. Tiny renal cysts noted in both kidneys.

Normal abdominal aortic calibre. No significant enlarged para-aortic, iliac or mesenteric lymphadenopathy demonstrated. No significant ascites demonstrated. No sign of pneumoperitoneum.

No gross small bowel or large bowel mass lesion demonstrated. The appendix appears normal. No evidence of colonic diverticulosis/diverticulitis.

There are multiple calcified lesions in the uterus which likely represent calcified uterine leiomyomas, the largest measures 2.75cm x 2.42cm x 3.26cm. No pelvic/adnexal mass lesion demonstrated. No pelvic focal collection or significant free fluid shown. The bilateral ischiorectal fossae are clear.

CONCLUSION:

There is an ulcer crater with enhancing mucosal thickening demonstrated in the gastric pylorus which likely represents the biopsy proven malignant gastric ulcer. It measures about 1.56cm x 2.45cm x 4.93cm in size. There is associated nonspecific gastric wall thickening extending into the distal pyloric antrum. No gross extra-luminal tumour infiltration of the perigastric fat or adjacent structure demonstrated. No significant regional enlarged lymphadenopathy demonstrated.

There are multiple well-defined hypodense hypoenhancing foci in both lobes of liver which may represent hepatic cysts, although cystic metastases from adenocarcinoma cannot be definitely excluded, the largest in the left lobe measures 1.66cm x 2.07cm x 1.54cm and the largest in the right lobe measures 1.08cm x 1.72cm x 1.63cm.

There are two nonspecific small nodules in the left lung base. No discrete focal lesion identified in the right lung base. No pleural effusion demonstrated.

C
T

S
C
A
N

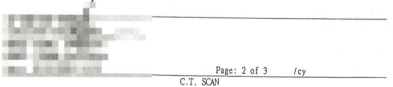

C.T. SCAN

↻ 2006 年 10 月 20 日检查报告显示幽门部溃疡性胃癌，确认了病理活检的诊断，肝脏有多发病灶，肺部也有两个结节病灶

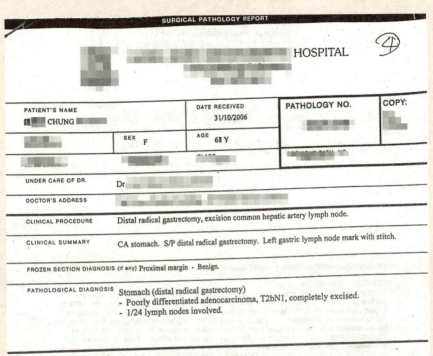

SURGICAL PATHOLOGY REPORT

HOSTPITAL

PATIENT'S NAME		DATE RECEIVED	PATHOLOGY NO.	COPY:
CHUNG		31/10/2006		
	SEX F	AGE 68 Y		

UNDER CARE OF DR. Dr.

DOCTOR'S ADDRESS

CLINICAL PROCEDURE Distal radical gastrectomy, excision common hepatic artery lymph node.

CLINICAL SUMMARY CA stomach. S/P distal radical gastrectomy. Left gastric lymph node mark with stitch.

FROZEN SECTION DIAGNOSIS (if any) Proximal margin - Benign.

PATHOLOGICAL DIAGNOSIS Stomach (distal radical gastrectomy)
- Poorly differentiated adenocarcinoma, T2bN1, completely excised.
- 1/24 lymph nodes involved.

REPORT

Supplementary Report

Immunostaining for cytokeratin shows infiltration of one distal greater curve lymph node, not seen on superficial levels of the paraffin block. The other lymph nodes, including the common hepatic artery lymph nodes, are negative.

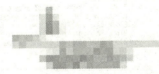

Date Reported: 04/11/2006

Ω 2006 年 10 月 31 日胃手术后病理学检查报告：胃低分化腺癌，有淋巴转移

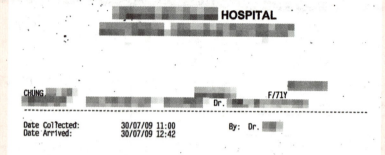

HOSPITAL

CHUNG   Dr.   F/71Y

Date Collected: 30/07/09 11:00   By: Dr.
Date Arrived: 30/07/09 12:42

Pathology Report

SPECIMEN TYPE
Right hemicolectomy.

CLINICAL DETAILS
Perforated appendiceal base + caecal tumour.

MACROSCOPIC EXAMINATION
Specimen received fresh and subsequently fixed in formalin with patient's data and designated colon. It consists of right colon, appendix and terminal ileum. The colonic segment measures 16 cm in length and 10 cm in maximum circumference at the caecum and 7 cm in maximum circumference at the ascending colon. The appendix measures 6 cm long and 1 cm in maximum diameter. The small intestine segment measures 35 cm long and 4 cm in maximum diameter. Outer surface of the colon, caecum and distal ileum is covered with inflammatory exudate. The appendix is dilated and covered with exudate. Small perforation is noted at the base of appendix. On opening, there is polypoid tan colored firm tumour at the caecum covering the appendiceal orifice, measuring 4 x 4 x 3 cm. It is 11 cm away from the distal resection margin and 35 cm from the proximal resection margin. The retro-caecal circumferential margin is inked blue, the perforation area is inked black and the rest of the serosal surface is inked yellow. Serial sections show whitish infiltrative tumour infiltrating the muscle coat and extending into the subserosal soft tissue, close to the perforation area. Multiple lymph nodes are identified in the mesenteric fat. The largest one measures 2 cm in maximum dimension. No soft tissue tumoral deposit is noted grossly.
Block 1 - proximal resection margin.
Block 2 - distal resection margin.
Block 3 - apical mesenteric resection margin.
Blocks 4 to 8 - tumour with the perforation area.
Block 9 - polypoid part of the tumour.
Block 10 - appendix.
Block 11 - circumferential margin (contain one lymph node bisected).
Blocks 12 to 14 - apical lymph nodes (blocks 13 and 14 - one lymph node bisected each).
Blocks 15 to 17 - caecal lymph nodes (block 17 - two lymph nodes, the largest is bisected).
Block 18 - lymph nodes of ascending colon.
Blocks 19 & 20 - ileal lymph nodes.
Block 21 - sampling of the small bowel.
Block 22 - sampling of the small bowel.
Block 23 - sampling of the caecum.

MICROSCOPIC EXAMINATION
Sections show a moderately differentiated adenocarcinoma forming cribriform and irregular angulated glandular pattern with focal mucin extravasation. The tumour shows moderate nuclear pleomorphism and hyperchromasia. Lympho-vascular permeation is not apparent. Adenomatous changes with low grade dysplasia is focally seen at the edge of the adenocarcinoma. Lymphoid reaction towards the tumor is mild. The tumor invades through

* Ward enquiry – screen capture   Page 1   to be continued...

HOSPITAL

CHUNG,   F/71Y
                                          Dr.

Date Collected: 30/07/09 11:00   By: Dr.
Date Arrived: 30/07/09 12:42

the muscularis propria. Serosa is not involved. Resection margins, including the apical
mesenteric, circumferential, proximal and distal margins are clear. Two out of 14
paracolic lymph nodes show metastasis. The 10 apical and 9 ileal lymph nodes are negative
for malignancy.
The perforation site at the base of appendix is noted and accompany with abscess
formation and inflamed fibrosing granulation tissue. No malignant gland is seen at the
perforation site. A sessile serrated adenoma is noted at the tip of appendix.

DIAGNOSIS
Right hemicolectomy:
-Moderately-differentiated Adenocarcinoma of cecum.
-Invades through muscularis propria.
-Serosa is not involved.
-Two out of 33 lymph nodes show metastasis.
-Resection margins are clear.
-pT3N1.
-Perforation at base of appendix with abscess and granulation tissue formation.
-Sessile serrated adenoma of appendix noted.

Pathology Report   Authorized By: Dr.   06/08/09 10:29
                     *** This Laboratory is NATA & RCPA accredited ***

                   ********** End of report **********

Report Destination:

∩ 2009 年 7 月 30 日肠手术后病理学检查报告：盲肠中分化腺癌，侵入固有肌层，
有淋巴转移。阑尾穿孔并有脓肿及肉芽组织形成

素食的好处

◇ 东西方文明的素食历史

在古希腊时代，著名学者苏格拉底、柏拉图、毕达哥拉斯都是素食主义的代表，他们认为素食才可以获取纯净的智慧，素食是"智慧者"的选择，并将素食主义风潮漫及整个古希腊。欧洲文艺复兴时代，米开朗琪罗、达·芬奇、莎士比亚、拉斐尔等伟大著名的代表人物都提倡素食，并将素食主义的传统作为"贵族"气息延续到了近代。伏尔泰、雪莱、萧伯纳、爱因斯坦、罗素等都是影响着近代史的伟大人物，也都是素食者并极力劝导他人食素。

中国素食的传统最早可以追溯到夏商时期。在《礼记》中有记载曰："逢子卯，稷食菜羹"，从初一到十五吃素，遂成习俗。至今，仍维持着初一、十五斋戒食素的习惯。《左传》中也有记载："肉食者鄙，未能远谋"。

古老的中医学一直强调清淡饮食，避免肥甘厚味。药王孙思邈在《备急千金翼方》中说："食之不已，为人作患，是故食鲜肴务令简少；故其鱼脍、生菜、生肉、腥冷物多损于人，宜常断之"。是讲一定要少吃荤食。至宋代，据《梦粱录》等古籍记载，已有上百种不同的花卉、药草、水果、豆类、豆腐制品等素食烹饪技巧。

◇ 素食的好处

其实肉食消耗越来越多的情况，也就是近代，或者说是近

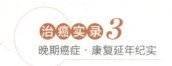

几十年才发展到这种程度的。相应的恶性肿瘤的发病率也在近几十年翻了几十倍。全世界如都以素食为主要食品，种植、养殖行业也会有巨大的转变，可使人类更加健康。

素食者培养了"慈祥、仁爱、尊重"的性格，更容易情绪稳定，心情平静，而自在而安详的心态可以预防形成癌症性格以及避免遭癌症的侵害。

综括而言，素食的好处有以下几点。

1.吃素减低患癌风险

食用大量新鲜蔬菜水果，可以大幅降低罹患肝癌、结肠癌、胰脏癌、胃癌、膀胱癌、子宫颈癌、卵巢癌等癌症的危险，大量食用蔬果的人比不常食用的人患癌概率减少一半！中国的研究也得出相同的结论：从1984年起，有关专家调查中国人生活习惯与癌症产生的关系发现，大量吃蔬菜者比起很少吃蔬菜的人，肺癌、结肠癌、直肠癌发生率均显著降低。

2.吃素有益脑血管

吃大量蔬菜水果可以降低心脏病和中风的发病率。在心脏病发之后，蔬菜水果也是一剂良药。美国白宫健康医疗顾问欧宁胥曾长期做过一项病理研究，他发现心脏病、中风患者要想成功恢复健康，就必须全面改变饮食结构，尽量少吃肉，以素食为主！

3.吃素能增强免疫力

英国畅销书《健康百分百》指出，要增强免疫力，专家的第一个建议就是每天多吃蔬菜水果。素食更有免疫优势。

4.吃素使身体强健

长久以来错误的观念——吃素没营养，是没有根据的！最高大的动物如牛、象、长颈鹿等都是吃素的！拳王阿里亦是茹素一族。另一种错误的观念是"吃素不聪明"，看看历史上素食的诺贝尔奖得主如泰戈尔、爱因斯坦等。其实，从古至今，无论是东方还是西方，都认为素食才是最聪明最有智慧的。

病案20

晚期卵巢癌多发转移，如今已度19年

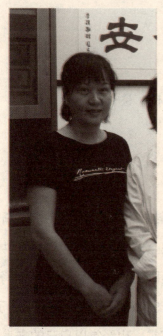

陈女士于1999年患卵巢癌做了手术切除，并把子宫及所有附件、大网膜等全切了。2006年肿瘤腹腔复发，她再次手术并化疗。此后她的病情逐渐加重，腹痛严重无法缓解，长期服用多种止痛西药，导致恶心、呕吐等多种副作用，疼痛却又越来越严重，腹部的肿瘤也越来越大。至2014年时医院已无法可医，腹腔转移肿瘤生长很快，已达9.6cm。陈女士因疼痛非常严重，属无药可医的晚期癌症而用上了吗啡，

🎧 陈女士于2018年7月来诊时留影

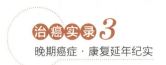

造成药物成瘾，用量越来越大，疼痛仍不能缓解。陈女士非常担心大量使用吗啡造成的各种副作用和成瘾性。

医生对她讲得很明白，这样的药物只能给予晚期无法治疗且生命非常有限的患者。而且因肿瘤很大，压迫造成了肛门坠重，疼痛难忍，大便难排，便感时时都有。陈女士不甘心就此逐渐衰弱离世，经多方打听，前来中心治疗。

通滞消瘤，破血逐瘀。

治疗方案

(1) 常用中药：香附、枳实、莪术、三棱、桃仁、红花、土鳖虫、白芍、当归、橘核等。
(2) 散结丸、化癥丸同时服用。

经生命修复治疗后，陈女士的精神好转，各种痛苦的症状逐渐减轻，以至消失，逐渐摆脱了吗啡成瘾，到完全停用吗啡，也治好了肿瘤造成的严重腹痛。长期因下坠感严重不能坐卧行走的症状，现在也消失了。腹腔中无法切除的肿瘤在2年多前已有9.6cm，现在逐渐摸不到了，但是还没有去医院检查。陈女士现在生活正常，也经常以自己的亲身经历鼓励其他患者，增强他们战胜癌症的信心。

附：患者相关检查报告

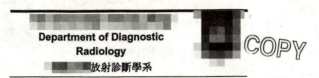

Department of Diagnostic Radiology

放射診斷學系

Name of Patient:	CHEN,		
Sex / Age:	F/36Y		
Our Centre Code:		**HKID:**	
Date Attended:	19/06/2014	**Date Reported:**	19/06/2014
Referring Dr.:			
Institution:			
Examination:			
Imaging No.:			

Blood Glucose Level Before F18-FDG Injection: 9.8 mmol/L
F-18 Fluorodeoxyglucose Injected: 10.4 mCi
F-18 Fluorodeoxyglucose Uptake: 1 Hour 0 Min
IV contrast: 90 mL   Iopamiro 370 injected at 2 mL/Sec

Whole body PET-CT

History :

Recurrent CA ovary with previous OT and multiple chemotherapy. Rising CA 125.

Imaging Technique :

Whole body FDG PET and contrast-enhanced 64-MDCT was performed from the base of the skull to the upper thighs.

Report :

Previous CT taken on 6/12/2012 is retrieved as reference.

Head and neck

From the base of skull to the thoracic inlet, there is symmetric, physiological distribution of activity with no focal areas of abnormal uptake demonstrated.
The imaged portion of the brain is unremarkable.

Chest

Lungs are clear without discrete hypermetabolic focus. There is no discrete nodule detected in the corresponding CT images.
Evaluation of the mediastinum reveals no hypermetabolic focus.

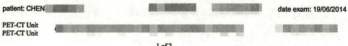

patient: CHEN   date exam: 19/06/2014

PET-CT Unit
PET-CT Unit

1 of 2

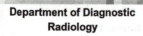

Department of Diagnostic Radiology

放射診斷學系

There is no pleural nor peri-cardial effusion seen.

Abdomen and pelvis

Multiloculated cystic lesion in the left lower pelvis is noted with mildly increased FDG uptake (SUVmax = 1.5).
It shows interval increase in size (longest dimensions = 9.6cm) and soft tissue component when compared to the previous CT.
Radiologically, features are suggestive of disease progression.

The lesion exerts mass effect onto the urinary bladder anteriorly.

The background FDG uptake of the liver is homogenous without discrete hypermetabolic focus. (SUVmax = 1.9).
Intra-hepatic and common ducts are not dilated.
The gallbladder, pancreas and spleen are unremarkable.
Bilateral kidneys are comparable in contrast excretion. Bilateral renal pelvis are slightly prominent.
Both adrenal glands are normal.
Evaluation of the para-aortic region reveals no hypermetabolic focus.
There is no ascites seen.

Skeletal system

Marrow uptake is unremarkable.
In the corresponding CT images, no osseus lesion is seen.

Opinion :

Multiloculated cystic lesion in the left lower pelvis with interval increase in size and soft tissue component. Radiologically, features are suggestive of disease progression.

patient: CHEN,   date exam: 19/06/2014

PET-CT Unit
PET-CT Unit

2 of 2

↷ 2014 年 6 月 19 日检查报告示：盆腔肿瘤增大，病情加重，肿瘤已有 9.6cm

抗癌常用中药

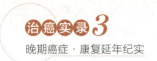
◇ 常用扶正中药

❋ 人参

人参味甘、微苦，性平。归肺、脾、心经。大补元气，复脉固脱，补脾益肺，生津，安神。适用于各种常见肿瘤证见气虚或虚脱者。

❋ 西洋参

西洋参又名花旗参，味甘、微苦，性寒。归肺、心、肾、脾经。主要成分为人参皂苷、挥发油、树脂等。能补气养阴，清火生津，养阴清热。

❋ 茯苓

茯苓味甘、淡，性平。归脾、心、肾经。具利水渗湿，健脾补中，宁心安神的功效。适用于各种常见肿瘤患者，有健脾利水之用。

❋ 当归

当归为伞形科植物，根为正品。味甘、辛，性温。归肝、心、脾经。当归具补血、活血、止痛、润肠通便的功效。适用于常见肿瘤有血虚体弱、疼痛眩晕等症。

❋ 绞股蓝

绞股蓝是葫芦科草质藤本植物，味苦、微甘，性凉。能化浊补虚，化痰解毒。用于常见肿瘤体虚乏力、痰浊咳喘等。

❋ 白术

白术味甘、苦，性温。归脾、胃经。补脾气，燥湿，利水，固表止汗。适用于常见肿瘤，健脾燥湿。

✳ 山茱萸

山茱萸味甘、酸，性微温。归肾、肝经。有补肾气，益肾精，固脱，敛汗，缩尿的功效。适用于常见肿瘤肝肾不足、汗多尿频等。

✳ 百合

百合味甘，性微寒。归肺、心、胃经。有清心安神，养阴润肺止咳的功效，适用于阴虚咳喘、心悸者，以及肺癌、淋巴肉瘤等阴虚者。

✳ 灵芝

灵芝为多孔菌科植物紫芝或赤芝的子实体。味甘，性平。益精气，养心安神，止咳平喘，滋养强壮，补虚抗癌。有安神补虚之用。

✳ 仙鹤草

仙鹤草味苦、涩，性平。归肺、脾、肝经。收敛止血，补虚，消积，杀虫。用于常见肿瘤有出血，眩晕，神疲乏力等。

◇ 常用解毒排毒抗癌中药

✳ 石见穿

石见穿味苦、辛，性平。归肝经。主要功效为清热解毒，活血化瘀。适用于食管癌、胃癌、肠癌及其他常见肿瘤有热毒症状者。

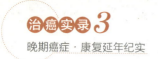

※ 石上柏

石上柏味甘，性平。归肺、肝经。主要功效为清热解毒、凉血止血。用于常见肿瘤有热毒、出血等症者。

※ 藤梨根

藤梨根味酸、涩，性凉。归胃、膀胱经。主要功效为清热解毒，祛风燥湿，消肿止血。用于消化道肿瘤及常见肿瘤。

※ 牛黄

牛黄味苦甘，性寒。归心、肝经。主要功效为清热解毒、镇惊、祛痰开窍、利胆。适用于常见各种癌瘤，如脑瘤、肝癌、肺癌、白血病等有热毒症状者。

※ 七叶一枝花

七叶一枝花又名蚤休、重楼。味苦，性微寒，有小毒。归肝经。主要功效为清热解毒、消肿止痛，息风定痉。多用于热毒壅滞的恶性淋巴瘤、肺癌、鼻咽癌、脑肿瘤及消化系统肿瘤如胃癌、食管癌、肝癌等。

※ 白花蛇舌草

白花蛇舌草味甘淡，性凉。归胃、大肠、小肠经。主要功效为清热解毒、软坚散结、利水消肿。适用于常见癌瘤及消化道癌瘤。

※ 白英

白英又名蜀羊泉。味苦，性微寒。归肝、胃经。主要功效为清热解毒、利水消肿。适用于常见肿瘤如肝癌、胃癌、肺癌、膀胱癌及宫颈癌等。

❋ 半枝莲

半枝莲味辛，性凉。归心、肺经。主要功效为清热解毒、利水消肿。适用于各类常见肿瘤。

❋ 龙葵

龙葵味苦，性寒，有小毒。归胃、膀胱经。主要功效为清热解毒、利水消肿。适用于常见肿瘤有热毒，水肿等症。

❋ 甘草

甘草为豆科植物甘草的根茎和根，味甘，性平。归心、脾、肺、胃经。主要功效为补中益气、泻火解毒、润肺祛痰、缓和药性、缓急定痛。

❋ 绿豆

绿豆为豆科植物绿豆的种子。主要功效为清热解毒、消暑。用于疮毒痈肿，排毒祛浊。

❋ 板蓝根

板蓝根为十字花科植物菘蓝的根，主要功效为清热解毒、凉血。用于清热解毒，凉血。

❋ 金银花

金银花为忍冬科植物忍冬的花蕾。味甘，性寒。主要功效为清热解毒、疏风散热、抗炎清热。

❋ 连翘

连翘为木犀科植物连翘的果实，主要功效为清热解毒，常与金银花同用。

❋ 猪殃殃

猪殃殃味辛苦，性凉。归脾、心、小肠三经。主要功效为

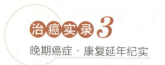
清热解毒、利尿消肿。对 S180 有抑制作用。适应证为肠癌、膀胱癌、肝癌、淋巴肉瘤、癌肿、白血病及乳腺癌等。

◇ 常用软坚散结抗癌的中药

✳ 山慈菇

山慈菇味辛，性寒，有小毒。归肝、胃经。主要功效为清热解毒、消肿散结。适用于乳腺癌、甲状腺癌、皮肤癌、恶性淋巴瘤等。

✳ 夏枯草

夏枯草味辛、苦，性寒。归肝、胆经。主要功效为清热泻火、软坚散结。适用于胃癌，甲状腺癌、乳腺癌、肝癌、恶性淋巴瘤等。

✳ 猫爪草

猫爪草味辛，性温、平，有小毒。归胆经。主要功效为解毒消肿，软坚散结。适用于常见肿瘤及甲状腺癌、乳腺癌等。

✳ 海藻

海藻味咸，性寒。归肝、胃、肾三经。主要功效为化痰散结、利水消肿。适用于甲状腺癌、胃癌、肝癌、肺癌及恶性淋巴瘤等。

✳ 昆布

昆布是海带科植物海带或鹅掌菜、裙带菜的叶状体。味咸，性寒。归脾、肝、肾经。主要功效为消瘀散结、利水消肿。

❋ 僵蚕

僵蚕味咸、辛，性平。归肝、肺、胃经。主要功效为息风止痉、祛风通络止痛、化痰散结。适用于脑瘤、肺癌、喉癌、常见肿瘤有淋巴结肿大者等。

❋ 牡蛎

牡蛎味咸、涩，性微寒。归肝、胆、肾经。主要功效为软坚散结、平肝潜阳、固涩制酸。适用于常见肿瘤及肺癌、肝癌、胃癌、甲状腺癌及恶性淋巴瘤等。

❋ 海蛤壳

海蛤壳味咸，性寒。归肺、胃经。主要功效为清肺化痰、软坚散结。

◇ 常用活血化瘀抗癌的中药

❋ 三七

三七味甘、微苦，性微温。归心、肝、脾经。主要功效为化瘀止血、活血消肿镇痛。主治各种出血证及跌仆瘀肿，胸痹肿痛。临床上常用治肺癌、食管癌、宫颈癌等癌瘤属瘀血阻滞或兼出血者。

❋ 䗪虫

䗪虫别名土鳖虫。味辛、咸，性寒，有小毒。归肝经。主要功效为破血逐瘀、续筋接骨。适用于常见肿瘤有气血瘀滞者及肝癌、宫颈癌、骨肉瘤及多发性骨髓瘤等。

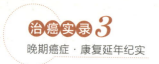

※ **丹参**

丹参味辛、苦，性微寒。归心、肝经。主要功效为活血祛瘀、凉血调经、养血安神。适用于常见肿瘤有血热、血瘀等症。

◇ **常用止痛抗癌的中药**

※ **姜黄**

姜黄味辛、苦，性温。归肝、脾经。主要功效为活血行气、通络止痛。适应证为肝、胆、胰头癌等气滞血瘀者。

※ **郁金**

郁金味辛、苦，性寒。归肝、胆、心经。主要功效为活血止痛、行气解郁、清心凉血、利胆退黄。适用于常见肿瘤及肝癌、胆囊癌、胰头癌等气滞血瘀者。

※ **威灵仙**

威灵仙味辛、苦，性微温。归肝、肾经。主要功效为祛风湿、通经络、止痛。适用于常见肿瘤以通经活络。

※ **白芍**

白芍味苦、甘、酸，性微寒。归肝、脾、心经。主要功效为补血柔肝、平抑肝阳、缓急止痛、敛阴止汗。对艾氏腹水癌细胞有抑制作用。适用于常见肿瘤有疼痛筋挛、肝胃不和、汗多血虚等症者。

※ **莪术**

莪术是姜科植物蓬莪术的根茎。味辛、苦，性温。归肝、脾二经。主要功效为破血祛瘀、行气止痛。对 S180、L615 肝癌实体型有抑制作用。适用于常见肿瘤有气滞表现者，如子宫颈癌、肝癌、胃癌、肠癌及甲状腺癌等。

◇ 常用化痰抗癌的中药

※ 天冬

天冬味甘、苦，性寒。归肺、肾、胃经。主要功效为补肺肾胃阴、清肺胃热、降肾火、止咳祛痰。适用于肺癌、胃癌及乳腺癌等肺胃阴虚者。

※ 射干

射干味苦，性寒。归肺、肝二经。主要功效为清热解毒、利咽消痰。适应证为喉癌、扁桃体癌、食管癌、咽喉癌、肺癌等。

※ 硇砂

硇砂味咸、苦、辛，性温。归肝、脾、胃三经，有毒。主要功效为消积、化痰、软坚。有细胞毒作用，并有利水祛痰作用。适应证为食管癌及贲门癌。外用为主。

※ 紫菀

紫菀味辛、甘、苦，性微温。归肺经。主要功效为化痰止咳。常用于肺癌。

※ 杏仁

杏仁为蔷薇科植物杏或山杏的果仁（种子）。味苦，性微温，有小毒。归肺、大肠经。主要功效为祛痰止咳、平喘润肠。常

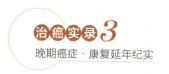

用于肺癌。

❋ 半夏

半夏味辛，性温，有毒。归肺、脾、胃经。主要功效为燥湿化痰、止咳、降逆、止呕、消肿散结、止痛。适用于常见肿瘤及宫颈癌、食管癌、胃癌、舌癌等。

◇ 常用利水祛湿抗癌中药

❋ 红豆杉

红豆杉味甘、苦，性平。主要功效为利尿消肿，通经化瘀。红豆杉又称紫杉，属国家一级保护的珍稀常绿乔木，枝、叶、皮、根可提取抗癌药物——紫杉醇。

❋ 薏苡仁

薏苡仁味甘、淡，性微寒。归脾、胃、肺经。主要功效为利水渗湿、健脾、舒筋、清热排脓。所含苡仁素有明显的抑制艾氏腹水癌的作用。适用于各种常见肿瘤有湿浊明显者。

❋ 苦参

苦参味苦性寒。入心、肝、胃、大肠经，主要功效为清热、燥湿、祛风、杀虫。对 S180、U14 及 EC 有抑制作用。适应证为宫颈癌、肝癌、大肠癌及皮肤癌等。

❋ 木瓜

木瓜味辛、酸，性微温。归肝、脾、胃经。主要功效为祛风、舒筋、化湿。适用于常见肿瘤，有健脾化湿之用。

❋ 泽泻

泽泻味甘、淡，性寒。归肾、膀胱经。主要功效为利水渗湿、泻热祛浊。

❋ 泽漆

泽漆味辛、苦，性微寒。有毒。归小肠、肺、大肠经。主要功效为利水消肿、化痰止咳，具抑瘤作用。适用于肺癌、肝癌及淋巴肉瘤等。

❋ 石韦

石韦味苦，性微寒。归肺、膀胱经。主要功效为利水通淋、清肺止咳、凉血止血。适应证为肺癌、膀胱癌及放疗、化疗后白细胞减少。

❋ 瞿麦

瞿麦味苦，性寒。归心、小肠、膀胱经。主要功效为利尿通淋、活血通经。适应证为泌尿系肿瘤。

❋ 猪苓

猪苓味甘、淡，性平。归肾、膀胱经。利水渗湿。对小鼠移植性肿瘤，腹水型肉瘤 –180 有明显的抑瘤作用。适用于常见肿瘤有水湿停滞的肺癌、膀胱癌、肾癌、前列腺癌等。

以上中药一定要在医生的辨证基础上开方使用，不可自己乱用。

中医药学的特色是辨证施治，生命修复治疗从人体生理、病理特点出发，自然会有相对应的理法方药，绝对不是抗癌药物或抗癌中药的堆积。脱离了辨证，即使把所有的抗癌药全放入一个药方中，也只能说是一个大杂烩，并不会有良好的效果。

晚期肠癌化疗失败，平安顺利已8年

叶太太于2009年感腹痛不适，2010年初因腹痛、血便去医院就诊，查出患肠癌，于2010年9月做手术。手术后病理学检查报告为直肠与结肠腺癌，并有大量淋巴转移，仅手术切除的肿瘤附带周围组织中，就有19个转移的淋巴结。

叶太太在做化疗时前来就诊，她开始时只是希望中医药能够减轻化疗的副作用。化疗中出现了呕吐、腹泻、皮疹、脱发，后来又出现肝、肾功能受损，全

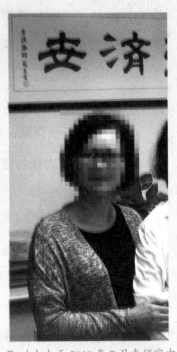

⚫ 叶太太于2018年7月来研究中心时留念

身疼痛、水肿、全血细胞减低等。以后西医又安排了靶向治疗、放射治疗等，在这些过程中增加使用中药的治疗，都起到了良好的作用，使她能够尽快从不良反应和毒副作用中得到恢复，以便进行下一个疗程的治疗。叶太太一直坚持治疗，希望这些西医的治疗结束后，转移的肿瘤能够消失。至2011年5月份已经做了多个疗程的化疗、靶向治疗及放射等治疗，但腹痛加重，

下肢水肿严重，经做 CT 检查，腹腔中有少数肿瘤缩小一些，但有更多的肿瘤却增大增多，腹腔肿瘤增大压迫阻碍下肢血液循环和回流，造成水肿、疼痛等。这时医生要求继续化疗，并增大剂量、改换药物种类等，但叶太太自感病情加重，治疗效果差，特别是又出现的一些新肿瘤和增大的肿瘤，使她失去信心，于是她自作主张停止了西医治疗如化疗、靶向治疗等，希望专用中医药治疗。

当时见她面色苍白、四肢无力、头晕耳鸣、恶心呕吐、便溏、便血、四肢水肿、冰冷无力，舌暗有瘀斑，脉细。

治疗原则

补正扶阳，化浊抗癌。

治疗方案

(1) 常用中药：制附片、地榆、槐角、马齿苋、守宫、茜草、桃仁、莪术、三棱、川大黄、猪苓、山药、薏苡仁、苍术等。

(2) 攻毒散同时服用。

患者湿盛阳亏，中气虚弱，气滞血瘀，癌毒势盛，治疗当补正攻邪，益气养血，畅达气机，消灭肿瘤。附子扶阳，地榆、槐角、马齿

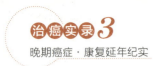

苋、茜草等凉血止血、解毒抗癌；三棱、莪术、川大黄、桃仁等化瘀、消滞攻积；猪苓、山药、薏苡仁、苍术健运中焦、祛湿益气。经过一段时间治疗后，她已没有任何不适，下肢严重肿胀已渐减退消失，身体逐渐康复。

2012年8月，医院报告显示，她的所有肿瘤全部消失，转移的淋巴结包括腹腔、腹股沟、腹膜后的淋巴结肿瘤也都全部消失。结果显示身体已没有任何肿瘤，健康正常。

在以后的中医药治疗中，叶太太遵循医嘱，持之以恒。时至今日，8年多已经过去了，叶太太仍坚持生命修复养生康复，也常常用自己的亲身抗癌经历鼓励患者和病友，告诉他们癌症不是绝症，癌症是可治的。

附：患者相关检查报告

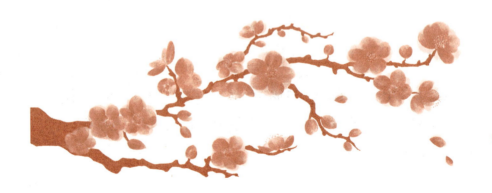

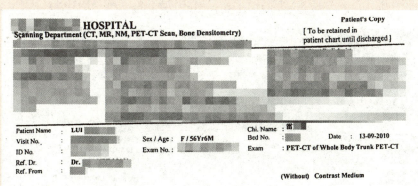

HOSPITAL
Scanning Department (CT, MR, NM, PET-CT Scan, Bone Densitometry)

Patient Name	: LUI			Chi. Name	: 雷		
Visit No.	:	Sex / Age :	F / 56Yr6M	Bed No.	:	Date :	13-09-2010
ID No.	:	Exam No. :		Exam	: PET-CT of Whole Body Trunk PET-CT		
Ref. Dr.	: Dr.						
Ref. From	:			(Without) Contrast Medium			

Clinical Information / History:

Newly diagnosed Ca upper rectum, 10 cm from the anal verge. For staging.

Blood glucose level is 5.6 mmol/l.

Radiological Report:

RADIOPHARMACEUTICAL:

9.1 mCi F-18 deoxyglucose.

FINDINGS:

Whole body trunk PET scan was performed from the base of skull to the upper thighs. Serial tomographic images of the whole body trunk were presented in transaxial, coronal and sagittal projections. Plain CT of whole body trunk was performed for image fusion with PET scan.

Intense abnormal uptake is demonstrated at the upper rectum, corresponding to the known primary cancer. Corresponding PET-CT demonstrates abnormal mural thickening. The lesion has a functional length of over 5 cm. SUV max = 9.25. Multiple hypermetabolic nodules are present at the perirectal, presacral and left common iliac areas. SUV max of these lesions are ranging from 3.0 to 4.0. These are most consistent with regional lymph node metastases. No significant lymphadenopathy is present at the paraaortic areas. The liver shows uniform physiological activity. Evidence of previous cholecystectomy is noted. No metachronous tumour is identified in the remaining large bowel.

No focal lesion is present in the head and neck and supraclavicular fossae. The upper aerodigestive tract is clear. There is no active lesion in the mediastinum and hila. No metastatic nodule is present in both lungs. Bilateral breasts and axillae are normal.

No focal lesion is present in the axial skeleton.

NO. OF FILMS	9	14" x 17"		(DDMM)	(HHMM)		
NO. OF COLOR PRINT	16	NO. OF CDR 1	'WET FILMS: SENT		REPORT & FILMS SENT OUT :		
Remark :			RETURNED		13-09-2010	PM OK	

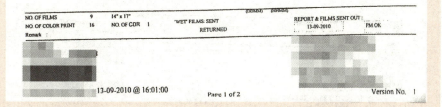

13-09-2010 @ 16:01:00   Page 1 of 2   Version No. 1

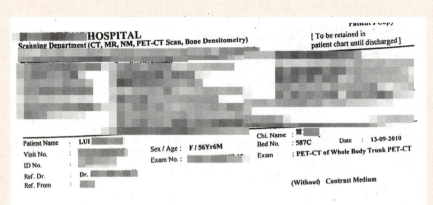

HOSPITAL
Scanning Department (CT, MR, NM, PET-CT Scan, Bone Densitometry)

[To be retained in patient chart until discharged]

Patient Name	: LUI	Chi. Name	: 雷
Visit No.	:	Bed No.	: 587C Date : 13-09-2010
ID No.	:	Sex / Age : F / 56Yr6M	
Ref. Dr.	: Dr.	Exam No. :	Exam : PET-CT of Whole Body Trunk PET-CT
Ref. From	:		(Without) Contrast Medium

(The plain CT images are performed for anatomical correlation and localization of lesion seen on PET. This is not a complete diagnostic contrast CT study).

(SUV = Standardized Glucose Uptake Value.)

IMPRESSION :

A primary cancer is present at the upper rectum. No metachronous tumour is identified in the remaining large bowel. Multiple metastatic lymph nodes are present at the perirectal, presacral and left common iliac areas. No suspicious lymph node is present at the paraaortic regions.

No distant metastasis is noted in the liver, lungs, bones and other organs in the entire body trunk.

Thank you for your referral.

(This examination does not include the brain.)

NO. OF FILMS	9 14" x 17"		(DDMM) (HHMM)	
NO. OF COLOR PRINT	16 NO. OF CDR 1	'WET FILMS: SENT	REPORT & FILMS SENT OUT : 13-09-2010	PM OK
Remark		RETURNED		

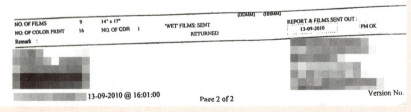

13-09-2010 @ 16:01:00   Page 2 of 2   Version No.

🎧 2010 年 9 月 13 日检查报告显示直肠上部肿瘤，有大量淋巴转移

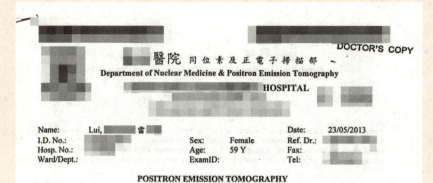

醫院 同位素及正電子掃描部
Department of Nuclear Medicine & Positron Emission Tomography
HOSPITAL

Name:	Lui, 雷	Date:	23/05/2013
I.D. No.:		Ref. Dr.:	
Hosp. No.:	Sex: Female	Fax:	
Ward/Dept.:	Age: 59 Y	Tel:	
	ExamID:		

POSITRON EMISSION TOMOGRAPHY
(^{18}F-FDG ONCOLOGY)

History:

A 59 year-old lady had laparoscopic resection of upper rectum in 09/2010, T3N2b disease, followed by chemotherapy and radiation therapy. PET here in 03/2011 showed mildly active nodes along right iliac vessel, aortocaval and paracaval regions. After 1 more cycle of chemotherapy, it was stopped due to side-effects. She switched to herbal medicine but later complained of right lower limb swelling. PET in 6/2011 showed improvement of myositis and nodes. She continued with herbal medicine. PET scan in 08/2012 showed no evidence of disease recurrence. Clinically asymptomatic. No further treatment was given. Hysterectomy for fibroid, cholecystectomy and appendectomy. Tumor marker found not useful for monitoring.

Radiopharmaceutical: 9.8 mCi F-18 Fluorodeoxyglucose (^{18}FDG) injected intravenously.

Findings:

Limited whole body CT transmission and PET emission imaging began at 60 minutes after radiopharmaceutical administration (blood glucose 5.2 mmol/l), spanning a region from base of skull to upper thigh. 60 mg Spasmonal was given p.o. 15 min before ^{18}FDG administration.

Liver tissue normal reference uptake has a SUVmax of 2.95.

Comparison is made with the prior study performed here in 08/2012. Patient is status post laparoscopic resection of rectal malignancy and radiation therapy. Surgery of the entire colon including the rectal suture shows no metabolic evidence of local recurrent disease. There is no hypermetabolic lymphadenopathy in bilateral groins, ischiorectal fossae, along iliac vessels or great vessels in the abdomen. The metastatic nodes in the retoperitoneum have subsided for 2 consecutive scans, in keeping with metabolic remission. No abnormal focal glycolysis in the omentum, mesentery, presacral regions and pelvic sidewall. There is no ascites.

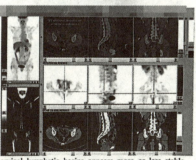

The small mildly active node in right upper cervical lymphatic basins appears more or less stable, suggestive of reactive node. Physiologic nasopharyngeal and thyroidal activity is present. In the thorax, there is normal parenchymal and pleural activity. The tiny nodule in inferolateral LUL remains stable and non active, suggestive of old granuloma. No hypermetabolic lymphadenopathy in bilateral hila and

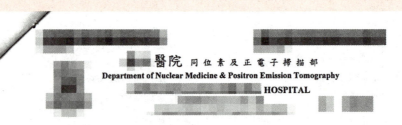

醫院 同位素及正電子掃描部
Department of Nuclear Medicine & Positron Emission Tomography
HOSPITAL

mediastinum. No pleural effusion. Bilateral axillae and breasts appear unremarkable. In the abdomen, there is normal size and metabolism in liver, spleen, adrenal glands and pancreas. No abnormal focal glycolysis in the stomach or the hysterectomy bed. Skeletal survey shows no hypermetabolic marrow activity to suggest active osseous metastasis. The myositis activities around bilateral hips are barely visible.

Impression:

1. No PET/CT evidence of local recurrence or regional metastatic lymphadenopathy given patient's history of treatment for rectal malignancy.
2. The hypermetabolic retroperitoneal nodes have subsided for 2 consecutive scans, in keeping with metabolic remission.
3. Stable reactive right upper cervical node and LUL tiny nodule.
4. No evidence of distant metastasis.
5. In summery: clinical remission.

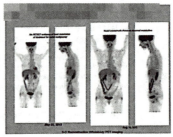

Thank you very much, Dr. ■ for your referral.

E544177 Lui Man Wai

🎧 2013 年 5 月 23 日检查报告显示转移病灶全部消失

多运动复健康

　　不少慢性病及肿瘤患者都会考虑用运动健身来强化体质，但应该根据个人生活方式、体能、年龄及日常消耗等因素，选择适合自身的锻炼项目和运动强度。

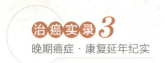

◇ 勿超负荷运动

　　许多患者会有长期挥之不去的持续疲劳感，可选择快步走或骑单车等锻炼。但是，锻炼身体时必须掌握好运动量，切不可超负荷运动。如果出现体温过高、病情复发或出血倾向、疲劳加重等都是不合适的。长期过度运动会损伤骨骼肌肉，增加心脑血管及心肺功能疾病风险，还会削弱免疫系统。

　　什么是"超负荷运动"呢？首先是自身的感觉，如果运动时出现轻度呼吸急促，感到有些心跳加快、周身微热，运动过后全身有轻松愉快的感觉，这表明运动适量；如果运动时呼吸困难、头晕目眩、大汗淋漓、心跳得像要蹦出来一样，运动过后全身沉重得不想再挪步，那一定是运动过度了。各种剧烈运动如快跑、爬山、打球、武术等过激运动都是不适合癌症患者的。

　　不同类型的肿瘤患者应当选择不同的锻炼方式，要因人、因病、因时制宜。肺癌患者可以通过均匀细长的腹式呼吸来改善肺功能。运动系统肿瘤（如骨癌）患者术后锻炼应以恢复运动功能为目的。胃癌、肠癌、肝癌等患者的锻炼则应以提高身体素质、减少疲劳为目的，通过适量运动改善消化功能。乳腺癌患者在术后更应早期进行肢体功能锻炼，尽快恢复患侧肢的关节、肌肉功能。

　　对于肿瘤手术患者来说，运动能避免其长期卧床造成肌肉萎缩、关节僵直或组织器官功能退化。如恢复良好，无禁忌证，散步、气功、太极拳或是做健身操、慢走等都是可行的选择。

而放疗、化疗之后的患者，如身体情况允许，应尽早开始养生活动，也很有帮助。

◇ **有氧运动和无氧运动**

近年来，有专家将锻炼方法分为有氧运动和无氧运动两类，前者指轻松的运动，肌肉不缺氧，后者指剧烈运动达到肌肉缺氧的状态。二者意义不同，后者可以提高肌肉的强度及耐力，有助于提高运动成绩，是运动员所追求的，而不是疾病患者应采用的。前者被科学试验证明，对于高血脂、糖尿病、高血压、心脑血管等疾病的康复和逆转有益。

对于慢性疾病、消耗性疾病及癌症患者，推荐使用太极拳运动。太极拳是中华民族特有的传统运动，适合癌症患者在治疗及康复中锻炼。很多患者放疗及化疗后身体处于极度虚弱的状态，所以应避免激烈的体育锻炼，选择柔和轻灵的太极拳锻炼是癌症患者康复期首选的好方法之一。

◇ **太极拳**

太极拳疗法是通过全身运动修复阴阳平衡来发挥作用的。太极拳讲究的是"形顺气自顺，气顺周身顺"，进而达到健身和养生的效果。太极拳运动在开合、虚实、动静中，以意导动，

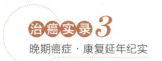
采气培元，快慢相间，刚柔相济。在练习中，讲究身体垂直中正，全身放松，呼吸顺畅，活动时不易感到疲劳，肌肉不会有酸痛、疲劳感。同时还能使唾液分泌增加，胃肠蠕动加快，可以及时清除人体废物及有毒物质，利于身体的康复。

太极拳动作柔和，锻炼后患者劳而不累，不仅利于肢体关节保健，还对胃肠道、肌肉神经以及大脑有保健作用，长期打太极拳可提高癌症患者身体免疫力，降低癌症复发危险。癌症患者的康复需要一个稳步恢复的过程，也要有良好的心态。打太极拳不仅锻炼了身体，也使身心得到极大放松，强化了自身免疫力，进而阻止和延缓了病程进展。通过太极拳慢慢调整人体的生理功能，从而增强体质，提高抗病能力，可以达到健身康复的目的。

◇ 癌症患者的气功锻炼

《黄帝内经·素问》讲："正气内存，邪不可干，精神内守，病安从来？"它告诉我们，气功锻炼有很好的防病治病作用，可以用作癌症患者的锻炼。

气功修炼遵循人与气互动循环的修炼模式，它一方面进行"心—身—形"协调统一的修炼——调心、调息、调身的"三调"锻炼，使人体精、气、神充足，内外气机协调一致，心理、生理、形态平衡，快速恢复精力和体力；另一方面，通过心身协调的平衡运动，增强体质，提高人体免疫力，促进心身健康。

实践说明，癌症患者当以练静功为主，动功为辅，也可动静交替练习，根据个人具体体质状态选择和制订适合的方案。

静功可选择放松功、松静功、打坐、吐纳功、内养功、五禽气功、站功、坐功和卧功等功法。

动功可选择八段锦、少林易筋经、简化太极拳等功法。

练功时注意选择环境宁静优雅、空气清新的地方，练功强度以适时、适度、愉悦为佳。

◇ 几点提示

首先，不要轻信别有用心的人打着气功的招牌过分夸大和吹嘘的一些毫不相关的活动，如特异功能、隔空取物等，这些与以健身康复为目的的气功锻炼是完全不同的。

其次，气功锻炼有相当严格的法则，如"轻松""虚静""自然"等为其基本要求。常见到有些人远离这些基本法则，将气功当作体育运动一样乱学乱做，这样反而会导致严重的损害身体和健康的后果。

晚期乳腺癌长寿之星

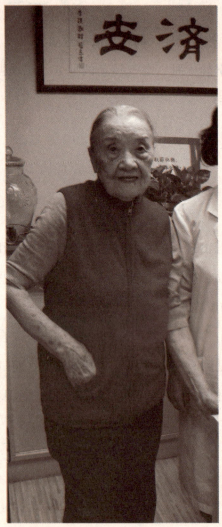

🔊 刘女士 2018 年 6 月前来就诊时，已 105 岁了，其在研究中心留影

如今人人谈癌色变，癌症给社会带来的危害毋庸置疑。患了癌症后，经现代化的医院治疗却英年早逝者不胜枚举。然而，也有很多的癌症患者包括晚期癌症患者却能够很好地生存下来。本书中所举的各个病案都是很好的例子，也是我们用生命修复的中医药治疗的成千上万的患者中的一些代表。为增强大家战胜癌症的信心，再举一位现已 105 岁的刘女士为例。

刘女士自幼生活艰辛，父母早逝，她有三个弟妹，自己是老大，从16岁就挑起了一家生活的重担，像母亲一样照顾弟妹，还要每天起早贪黑，种着几亩田地，养活一家大小。那时常常全家人吃了上顿没下顿，时常忍饥挨饿。一家人的衣食住行的生活重任全由她一人担当。夜半时分，也常常在昏暗的油灯下缝补衣服，大半辈子都是这样受苦过来的。70来岁时，才过上了舒适的日子，因为儿子在香港的公司生意做得越来越好，女儿也嫁了富裕人家。刘女士在儿子家住，也时常去女儿家闲住几日，无忧无虑。

但是世事难料，在刘女士近80岁时，准备好好享受老来福时，却查出患了乳腺癌并已有淋巴转移。在儿子的安排下，她先在医院做了手术切除肿瘤，然后第二步要进行化疗和放射治疗。刘女士住进了医院准备化疗和放射治疗时，看到同病房的患者在做化疗等都非常痛苦，脱发、呕吐、不能进食，也有人虽然经受了这些痛苦，但依然不能治好而离世。刘女士感到很害怕，但又知道与儿子女儿是无法商量的，他们一定会坚持要做这些治疗。

思前想后，最终在半夜时分自己擅自跑出医院，回到家里，以后无论谁来劝说，也不去医院了。这样在家里不做治疗的日子过了一年多，她胸部的皮肤有些地方发硬，成为一块一块的硬结。去医院检查的结果是乳腺癌皮肤皮下组织转移，淋巴转移，已经是晚期。刘女士还是不愿去做化疗等治疗。但是当听说有生命修复治疗时她很有兴趣，很快就前来进行中医药的治疗。那时她精神疲惫，瘦弱不堪，上肢水肿，胸部皮肤有溃烂。治疗以通经破滞、养肝败毒为主。

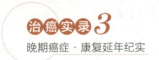

治疗原则

通经破滞，养肝败毒。

治疗方案

(1) 常用中药：当归、白芍、炮穿山甲、露蜂房、丹参、郁金、香附、鳖甲、王不留行、猫爪草等。

(2) 化癥丸同时服用。

经过约半年治疗后，刘女士的皮肤恢复正常，三年后结节均消失，气色好转，食量很好，体重增加。以后她间断地前来治疗，也一直坚持养生保健，她说现在虽然已 105 岁了，但精神比年轻时还好。

她现在愉快、健康，是当之无愧的抗癌长寿之星。

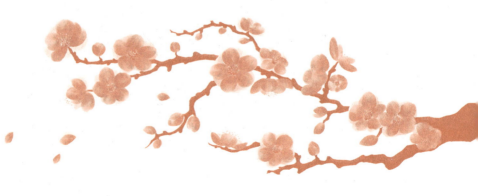